Lucky's Way

TURN YOUR
A**HOLE DOG
INTO AN ASSET

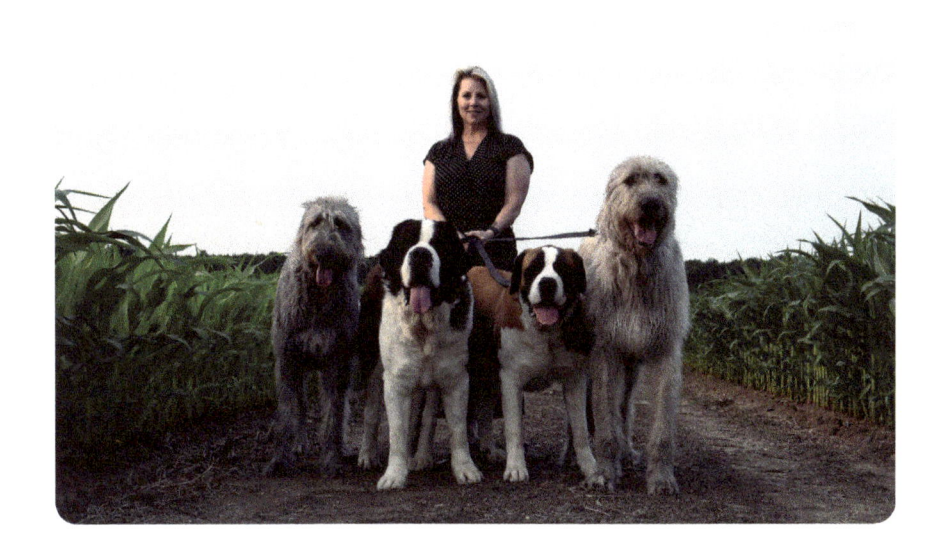

Brenda Boemer-Groenestege

◆ FriesenPress

Suite 300 - 990 Fort St
Victoria, BC, V8V 3K2
Canada

www.friesenpress.com

Copyright © 2020 by Brenda Boemer-Groenestege
First Edition — 2020

All rights reserved.

No part of this publication may be reproduced in any form, or by any means, electronic or mechanical, including photocopying, recording, or any information browsing, storage, or retrieval system, without permission in writing from FriesenPress.

ISBN
978-1-5255-5505-3 (Hardcover)
978-1-5255-5506-0 (Paperback)
978-1-5255-5507-7 (eBook)

1. PETS, DOGS

Distributed to the trade by The Ingram Book Company

For my Dad,
May every smile my dogs bring to others reach you in heaven.

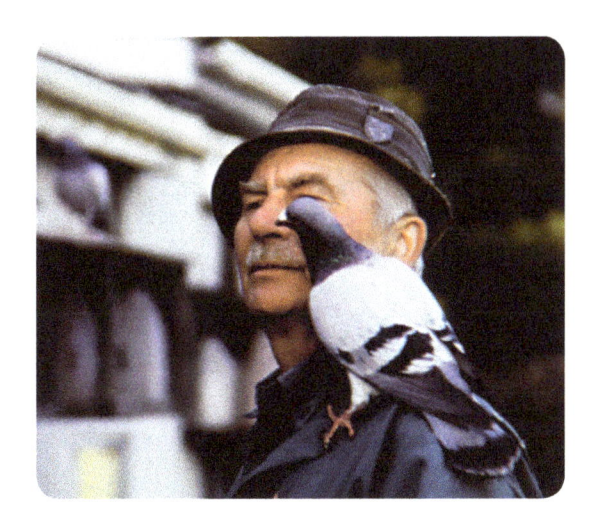

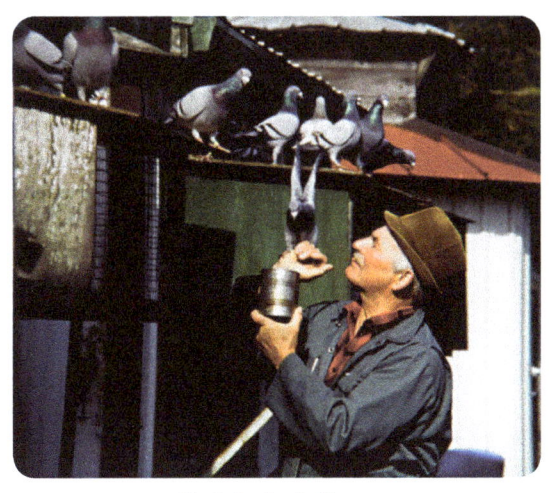

My dad... Lucky Boemer

TABLE OF CONTENTS

Forward vii
Introduction. xiii
Chapter 1: In the Beginning...Dad Introduced Me to the Dog 1
Chapter 2: My Therapy Dogs...and My Very Own A**hole Dog too! 13
Chapter 3: The Bond Between Father and Daughter...and Dog 25
Chapter 4: The Bonds We Make 37
Chapter 5: Making the Right Choices 43
Chapter 6: And So the Training Begins 81
Chapter 7: Train Your Dog to Become a Therapy Dog 115
Chapter 8: Frequently Asked Questions 121
Chapter 9: Lucky's Way...Tips You Won't Find In a Book or on Google 139
Chapter 10: Stories and Pictures from GG Therapy Dogs 163
Chapter 11: All Good Things Must Come To an End 181
Chapter 12: Pets Make Us Better People 193
Acknowledgments 195
Special Thanks. 199

FORWARD

Lucky's Way...
*Turn Your A**hole Dog into an Asset*
A guide to training your dog the easy way...

People constantly ask me the same two questions.

First, they ask me how I got into training and working with therapy dogs, and second, they ask if I've trained my own dogs because of how well-behaved they are when we go out to work on our dog therapy days.

The answer to question number one is easy. I got into dog therapy because of my parents. My father, Lucky Boemer, instilled in me—from a very young age—a deep-rooted love and respect for dogs. When I was growing up with them and him, he taught me his training methods and techniques, which I've come to appreciate and hone over the years, the more I work with and train dogs.

I guess that just answered question number two, right? Just to clarify, though, yes, I do train my own dogs. I'll touch on that a little later on.

As far as the a**hole part of this book, as soon as anyone hears that I train dogs, the first comment they make to me is, "My a**hole dog does _____. Can you help me?" or "I have an a**hole dog that does _____. How can I train it to stop?"

It's truly remarkable how many a**hole dogs seem to be out there, according to their owners, of course. Now, if I'm being honest here, and I promise I am, I also have a**hole dogs in my own family. Yes, you read that correctly, I, Brenda Henrietta Boemer-Groenestege the first (and yes, that is really my middle name...), have not only one, but two a**hole dogs living with me while I'm writing this book.

The first one is my superstar, Harold. I know, I know, that sounds like an oxymoron, calling him a superstar and then an a**hole, but I have to lay it all on the line here. And what exactly does this superstar a**hole do? He scratches at the door when he wants to come back into the house, but then just stands there and looks at you in the open doorway. Yup, that's my superstar a**hole dog. Now, you're probably thinking, "Come on, Brenda, that doesn't sound that bad," right? How would you feel if I told you he carries on this way sometimes for upwards of an hour or more?! Add to that, that it happens at all hours of the day and night! Yeah, that's not too annoying.

So, how do I deal with this? The obvious answer is to bribe him to come in with a treat. That's how I started doing it, and it definitely gets the wanted results; however, I DO NOT reward bad behaviour. Therefore, I pretend that he's going to get the cheese slice, and when he comes into the house, I give him praise, put the cheese slice back into the fridge, and go back to whatever I was doing. Now, if he comes in immediately, he gets lots of love and praise and the occasional treat.

On to a**hole number two...Clark Griswald. Oh my pearly pyjamas! Thank goodness Clark is as adorable as he is, or I'm not sure what would happen to him! Since he's the baby of the family, he seems to think he can get away with more, let's say, ridiculous behaviour. (I should know, I'm the baby in my family too!)

First, one of Clark's quirks is to be vocal when we're out at pet therapy. It's the strangest thing: I'll be talking, answering questions and whatnot, and all of a sudden, Clark starts barking at me. Just like that, out of the blue, barking. He'll be lying down comfortably by someone in the group therapy session and suddenly he feels the need to add his ten cents worth. Okay, I have to admit that it really is quite funny and our therapy friends get a complete hoot out of it, but I just wish I knew why he does it. He's probably just telling me to shut up!

Another thing Clark does, or rather, in this case, doesn't do, is get up to leave! Group therapy will be over, and I'll give the command, "Let's go, boys," and my other three jump up to follow me, but not Gris...nope, he just keeps lying there, with no intention of leaving. I'll walk up to him and nudge him with my foot and say again, "Let's go," and in response he'll flip over onto his back and want a full belly rub! Again, everyone in the room laughs and thinks that he's hysterical except me, because I know that what Clark wants is to be carried out, which is what I did when he was a puppy, but that's not happening now that he's a whopping 185 pounds of complete goofball!

Clark will eventually get up on his own when I decide to just leave with the other three dogs. Then he'll get up and run to catch up with us. This did bite me in the butt once, though, when I decided to leave him behind. A very sweet lady in a wheelchair didn't realize that I was leaving him on purpose, knowing that he'd eventually follow, and she grabbed his leash. You can imagine the ride she got that day, right?! Thankfully, she only got pulled about five feet before I turned around and saw what was happening. By the way, she loved every second of it!

I started the pet therapy part of my life after my mom had a stroke. We would visit her at her new senior living community on "Pet Visiting Days." Mom would ask me to bring in my dogs, which I, of course, happily did...I love showing off my dogs.

When I walked into the senior living community with two Saint Bernards, Truman at 185 pounds and Lloyd, still a puppy and therefore only weighing around 130 pounds, let's just say we got a lot of attention...at least Truman and Lloyd did. That was when I realized that there was actually a need for giant breed therapy dogs. The light bulb went on over my head after a gentleman lovingly pounded on Truman's side, saying, "Now this is a dog! The womenfolk, they like them their little dogs, but this big guy, well, he's what I call a real dog! We had one almost like this on our farm before we moved into town. Yeah, you're a good ole boy, aren't ya? Why, I don't even have to bend over to pet you. Good boy!"

It was a revelation. I started to really pay attention to Truman and Lloyd and how they were interacting with all the seniors. I saw how happy they were making them by just being themselves. It was absolutely incredible.

That's when my researching journey of how to train my own therapy dogs began. I had to break the news to my husband, Bob, that we were going to get a new puppy! He was not nearly as excited as I was about the prospect of another dog. Oh well, I was on a mission! Nothing, and no one, could stop me.

And so it began, with the choosing of a puppy.

I'm going to share my journey with you, which includes some of my favourite stories about my dad and his German shepherd, Asta, and, of course, my own experiences with my past dogs, as well as with my current GG Therapy Dog Team.

The GG is short for Gentle Giants. Harold and Leonard are my Irish Wolfhounds, and Lloyd and Clark are my Saint Bernards. We go into nursing homes, hospitals, schools, senior communities, local doctors' offices, and so many more places just to bring people joy.

In the following chapters, you will learn everything from how to pick the puppy best suited to your family, to how to find that perfect shelter pup, to how to go about training either dog to become a bombproof therapy dog...if that is your goal. Most people only want to have an amazing, mannerly, socialized, and well-behaved family pet.

I am also sharing with you my personal foolproof remedy for getting the skunk smell off your dog if it has been sprayed, along with other tips and tricks that I've picked up in my fifty-two years on this earth being around my dad and having him guide me with these amazing animals.

I will warn you, though, I speak quite frankly and honestly, and I'm not going to apologize for that. At the end of the day, I'm actually educating you, the human, the handler, about how to be the best, most confident, and most well-informed pet owner possible, which will result in you having a well-trained, well-behaved, well-socialized, and happy dog.

Ellen Degeneres ends every show with *"be kind to one another,"* a beautiful sentiment that I try to live my life by, while attempting to do my own personal favourite thing... I call this "ARK", which is short form for an "Act of Random Kindness"

So please everyone…

…do one ARK every day; it really is good for your soul.

Thank you, Brenda

Lucky's Way

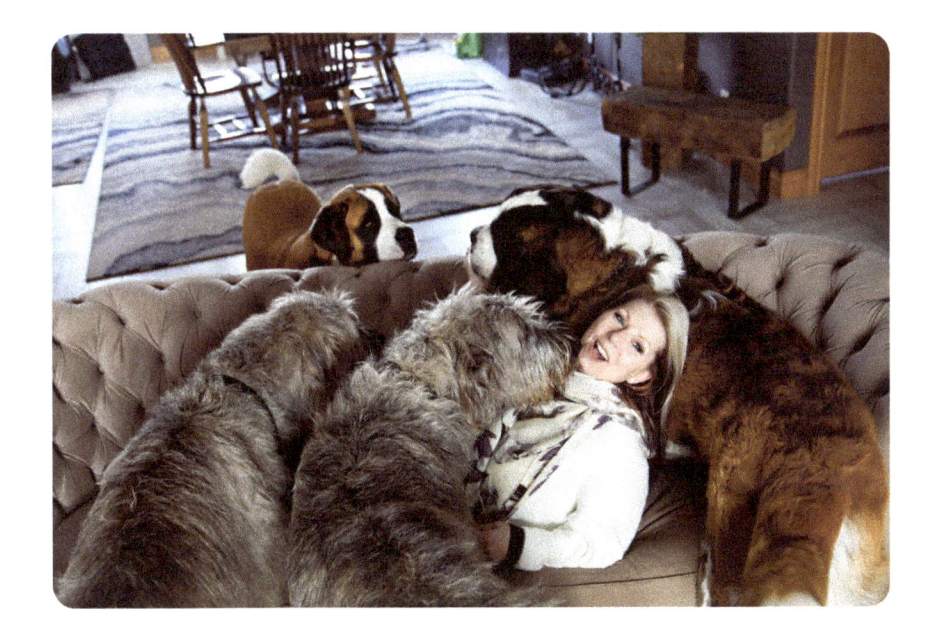

INTRODUCTION

My father, Lucky Boemer, trained German shepherds and worked with the police department in Germany before he came to Canada in the 1950s.

Now, some of his methods were pretty rough, but most of them were necessary because of the breed and temperament of the dogs. In Germany, they used what was considered "old blood" breeding methods, where they bred the bitch/female shepherd with a stud or male wolf. . I believe that, to this day, some breeders still use this same breeding methods to ensure the purest bloodlines and breeding stock..

That is why a male German shepherd, born and bred in Germany, fully matured, would weigh approximately 25–35 kg (55–77lb) and be approximately 55–65 cm (22–26 in) at the shoulder, with a deep slant in his hind end. Females would weigh approximately 20–30 kg (44–66 lb) and stand approximately 47–57 cm (19–22 in) at the shoulder, again, tapering to a steep slant in the hind end.

Because of this breeding, some of these pups grew up with enormous "attitude." That's where my dad came in. He knew how to train this type of dogs, and thankfully he shared a lot of that training with me before he passed away suddenly in 2002.

In my eyes, my father was an amazing man and it's an honour and a privilege to dedicate this guide to him, as well as to my mom, my kids, Spencer, Dylan, and Brooklyn, and my husband, Bob.

I decided to add real stories so you'd get a sense of who I am and how I came to train not only my own dogs, but help train other people's dogs as well. I want to share my love of these beautiful animals with you, so you can understand why they are so important to me and have played such an integral part in my life, not only today, but continuously throughout my past.

I will also share some of the stories my dad told me about his amazing dog Asta, who, by the way, still holds records in Germany. She shares a memorial wall, along with my father, in his hometown in Greven, at their local German shepherd club.

I could sit for hours and listen to story after story about my dad and never be bored. I miss him every day and wish that he was here to see what I've accomplished with my life, and especially with my dogs. Everything I do is just my way of paying tribute to him.

I love regaling my husband, my kids, oh heck, I love telling whoever's within earshot, some of the crazy things that my dad did that didn't even necessarily involve dogs. Just to give you some insight into my father's sense of, well, let's just call it his sense of humour, because *he* really thought what he was doing was funny and now, after the fact, I can sit back and laugh about it too, here is one of my all-time favourites.

DATE NIGHT DISASTER

My dad was a hunter and he took great pride in his collection of hunting rifles, which he would clean at the kitchen table…on date nights, conveniently, with our faithful poodle, Dusty, lying by his feet.

One night, when I was sixteen years old, I was anxiously waiting for my date to pick me up to go out for dinner and then to the drive-in movie theatre (for those who don't know what that is, it's an outdoor movie theatre where you sit in your vehicle and watch the movie on a big outdoor movie screen. The speaker hooks onto your window…oh heck, just google it).

Anyhow, my date pulled in the driveway and did the unthinkable, in my dad's eyes! *He honked the horn!* Yes, he did, and I guess he thought I was just going to come running out to him. But *that* sure didn't happen! Dusty was barking his brains out, which made things worse by the second.

"Please, Dad, just let me go outside," I pleaded.

"No vay!" my dad said angrily in his thick German accent. "No vone honks vur vone of mine daughters!"

Lucky's Way

So I waited while my date decided he would try honking again before eventually giving up and coming to the door. He was greeted by a yappy poodle and me, his hesitant date.

"Hey," he said at the door, "I honked, like, two times. Didn't you hear me?"

"Oh, I heard ya," I said, giving him a sympathetic look as I backed up and asked him to come in for a minute.

We walked into the kitchen and I introduced him to my mom first; he was still all smiles. Then I turned him around and, giving my dad one more pleading look, I introduced him to my rifle-cleaning, less-than-impressed dad.

At this point I noticed my date's smile begin to waver. I could tell he was trying desperately to be brave as he scanned the table and the heavily armed man in front of him. He stuck out his chest, stood up nice and straight, and confidently held out his hand, thinking to impress my dad with a manly handshake. He was greeted with a steely stare instead.

"You ever bin shot?" my dad asked him gruffly.

"Excuse me?" He stumbled back, not really understanding what my father was saying.

My dad gave him a good long hard stare with his steel-grey eyes and asked him again, "You ever been shot?"

"Umm, no," my date stammered. His face had begun to turn a deep shade of red, from his continuously moving Adam's apple right up to the very top of his perfectly feathered sun-kissed brown bangs.

As his hand, still empty, hung there in midair, my date slowly turned to me for some sort of guidance, and my dad snarled at him, "Honk fur mine daughter vonce more and I'll shoot you right in de ass!"

Well, I've never seen a face that went from crimson red to stark white so fast in all my life as I did that day! Since he was frozen on the spot, I grabbed him by the arm, said goodbye to my parents, and took off out the door. Dusty was hot on his heels, barking incessantly while I pushed my date outside.

As we left our house, he asked me if my father was always so "intense." I kind of laughed it off and told him that he was just a little protective, that's all.

xv

Unfortunately, the full colour never did return to my date's face, at least not in the entire half hour that our date lasted. Yeah, no dinner, no drive-in movie, no goodnight kiss, not even a hearty handshake at the door when he said goodnight to me! Nothing! He did, however, manage to walk me to the door. It seemed he was suddenly feeling gentlemanly enough to do that, but not feeling well enough to continue our date. Oh well, certainly not the right guy for me if he could be scared away that easily, right?

When I got home, my dad was watching TV. "Thirty minutes, Dad, that's a new record. Are you really going to do this every time I have a date?" I said.

Dad just gave me that grin. I didn't let him see it, but I was grinning too, behind his back.

Word spread like wildfire at my high school after that fiasco, and man, did my dating life go downhill fast! Pretty sure that was my dad's ultimate goal. God, I miss my dad… and I definitely miss that grin!

My dad with that grin!

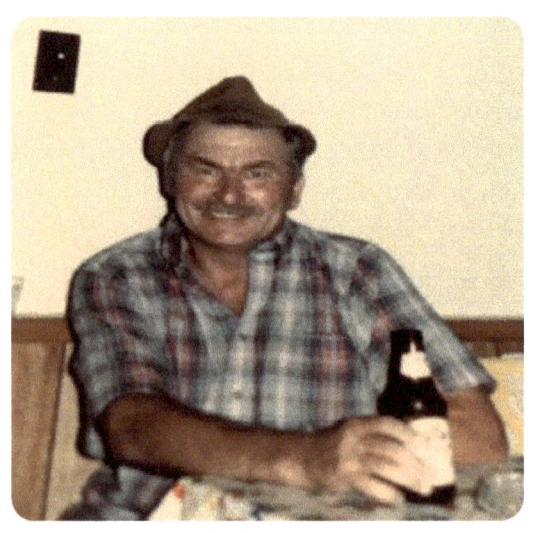

Lucky Boemer

CHAPTER 1

In the Beginning...Dad Introduced Me to the Dog

WHO PICKS WHOM?

It was my father who taught me that the best dog will be the one who picks you. Now, my dad also told me that the only good cat was the one who could swim when they were born (yikes)...oh, the stories I could tell you there! Better not.

Let's start at the beginning of my life with dogs. As far back as I can remember, we always had beagles. We would breed them, train them, and then sell the puppies to all of my dad's hunting friends. That was my first job and how I made my first money. If memory serves me correctly, we sold the males for $20 and the females for $25. What a deal, eh?

My dad was a big-time hunter and he loved our beagles. Thankfully, so did a lot of his hunting friends. They kept us busy and in the beagle breeding business for quite a while.

I certainly didn't mind. I loved those dogs. They were my best friends growing up. You see, I am the youngest of five kids, and we lived on the outskirts of the city. I didn't have any friends my own age nearby, so the dogs were always my go-to friends.

My mom tells stories of when I was a little girl; I would go missing, and my brother and sisters would notice the dog kennel door latched funny. Someone would check it out and there they'd find me, fast asleep in the dog house with the hounds. Funny thing is, I'm still sleeping with the dogs these days. Oh well, if it ain't broke, right?

Thankfully, I eventually did find some human friends and in grade six I found my best friend—like, really, really best friend. Her name is Julie. She's the yin to my yang, the peanut to my butter, the ice cream to my cake…you get it, right? We've been through hell together, and came out the other side laughing our fool heads off! The fact that she ended up marrying my brother Joe along the way put the cherry on top of the proverbial friendship cake.

Julie works at our local hospital, and quite often she will get approached by a coworker who asks, "Are you really related to Harold the therapy dog?" to which she very proudly replies, "Why, yes, I am, I've known him since before he was even famous!" I love the fact that Julie is as proud of my dogs as I am.

One day, after hearing about a really horrific motor vehicle accident with multiple deaths, I was talking to Julie and saying to her that I feel helpless when something like that happens in our little city. It really touches so many people. But what can you do?

Julie said, "I know how traumatized the staff is at the hospital. We don't handle these kind of accidents on a regular basis, so when they happen, it hits everyone really hard. I think they would really appreciate a visit from your therapy dogs in the emergency department. Even just for a few minutes to decompress…you know? The way that Harold and Leonard help people?"

I hadn't even thought of that. I go regularly to almost all the other departments in the hospital, but I just never gave a thought to going to emerge.

"Thanks, Jules, that's a great idea!" I said, and off we went.

The staff in emergency were so grateful! The hugs and squeezes that Harold and Leonard received that day, and the healing that they gave, were just phenomenal. Now when I go to the hospital, I started in the emergency department and work my way through the other departments.

Thanks to my BFF Julie, the entire staff and the patients at Stratford General Hospital get regular dog therapy from GG Therapy Dogs.

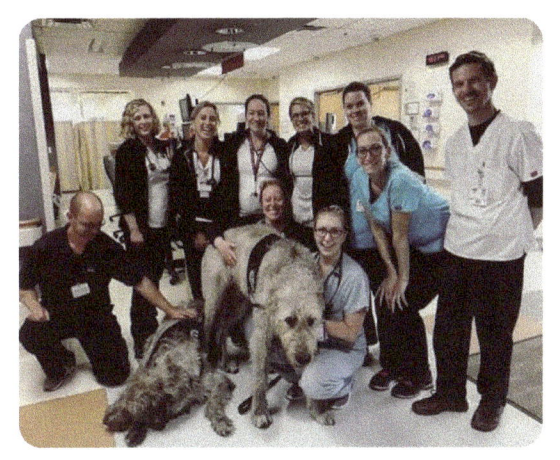

Harold and Leonard with Stratford Hospital staff

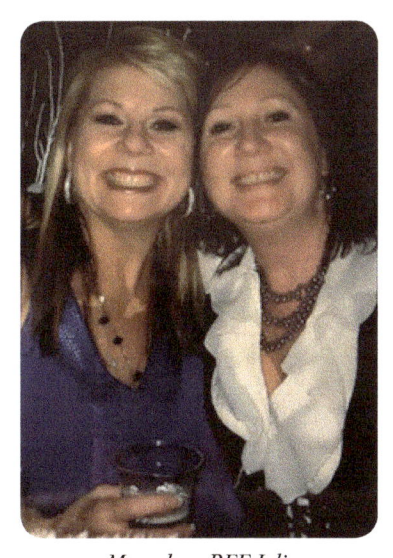

Me and my BFF Julie

MY GIFT WITH DOGS

My favourite story, as told by my parents, is one from when I was three years old. Every year we would all attend the annual summer pigeon party, and no, it's not a bunch of pigeons partying! It's a bunch of men who race homing pigeons on a weekly basis, which can actually be quite lucrative, if your pigeon comes home the fastest.

It's quite a fascinating hobby if you're at all interested in pigeons. My father was quite well-known for his birds and…oh shoot, forget the damn birds, this is about the dogs! Onward with the story…

So, we were all at this summer pigeon party pig roast (say that ten times fast), and there were lots of kids running around playing games, as well as men getting drunk and talking about their pigeons while watching the pig turning over and over again on the open spit of the fire. The ladies were all gathered together talking about whatever ladies talked about back then. It was the early seventies, so they were probably complaining about their kids and husbands, which is exactly what we women talk about now when we're together, right?

The people at this particular location happened to have a really vicious German shepherd tied up to their garage. They had BEWARE OF DOG signs everywhere and had warned everyone to stay away from the dog. You could see the boundary line where the dog's chain ended because the entire ground surface area had been completely worn down by the dog.

Of course, there were a couple of rotten little buggers who decided to taunt the dog by throwing sticks at him so the dog will try to chase them. They would get yelled at by the owners of the dog and their parents would get ahold of them and whack them with the same stick they were taunting the dog with. Ah, the good old days, when you could still whack your kids for being rotten without anyone looking down on you or calling children's aid (wink, wink).

The kids decided to get a soccer game going, and, as per usual, I was too young to play with them. It sucked always being the youngest.

Back then soccer wasn't like it is now, with parents actually paying constant attention to their children and making sure everyone is following the rules. Heck no! It was every kid for themselves! Which led to some very sore losers on the non-winning team! Mix sore losers with no parental guidance and you've got yourself a rotten little bugger looking to cause trouble. How did he accomplish this? He deliberately kicked the ball so hard it landed right over where the dangerous German shepherd was.

Well, of course that started a huge fight. Which finally got the adults' attention and the blame game began. Who was going to attempt to go over and retrieve the ball?

"You kicked it, you get it!"

"I'm not getting it!"

"You have to get it!"

"NO, you get it!" And so on and so on.

My mom said that that was when one lady stood up, shaking so badly she couldn't speak. She had placed one hand over her mouth and was pointing the other in the direction of the dog. Of course, all the ladies looked over to where she was pointing. As my mother described it, the lady let out a huge gasp and my mother told her to shut up and not say a word!

Mom said she looked over to my dad and just the look on her face had him coming over to see what was going on.

You could have heard a pigeon fart it was so quiet there. No one said a word. They all held their breath in complete amazement at the sight before them, including the owner of the dog, who wanted to go over, but my dad stopped him.

Apparently, here I was, over beside the German shepherd, kneeling down and petting him, kissing him and hugging him, before I grabbed the ball and started walking back to my siblings. That "mean" German shepherd did nothing to me. He accepted me as much as I accepted him. You see, unlike everyone else, I couldn't read yet. I had no idea about the Beware of the Dog sign.

Mom said it was only after I was out of reach of the dog that everyone began to breathe again. She had been so scared but apparently Dad said that he knew all along that the dog wouldn't hurt me (big eye roll from the women reading…because that's such a typical man response!). He explained that he'd known I've always had a gift with dogs and this just proved it. I personally don't remember this event, but I love hearing the story told.

It brings up a good question, though. Is it possible for some people to have a "gift" with dogs? Like my father said? I'm not sure if it's a gift or just a deep-rooted love, respect, and appreciation for them that I have. Either way, I will always have a dog in my life, of *that* I am *sure*. They keep me grounded. They keep me sane when my world is spinning off its axis.

Even as a child, when I was upset, it was my dogs who comforted me, who understood me. That is something that never stopped or changed over the years.

After my first serious heartbreak as a teenager, I was devastated and thought my life was over because my one true love, my soul mate, my reason to live and breathe, Jeff, broke up with me…sigh. I really thought he was "the one," like *the one,* the only one, and I would never, ever love again, like ever!! I was completely devastated!

It was only my dog Dusty, our miniature poodle, who understood what I was going through. I cried into Dusty's soft furry black neck for hours, thinking I'd never love again.

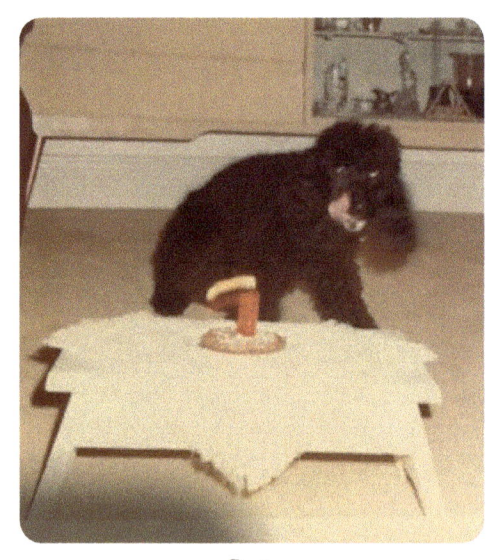

Dusty

I'm sure quite a few of you out there can relate to that, right? Funny thing, I did survive…but I still use the same method to soothe myself when I'm really upset.

When my dad died suddenly from a stroke, it was my dogs who caught my tears every night for months…actually, years, if I'm being honest here. I miss my dad every day. There's not one day that goes by that I don't think about him and wonder if he can see what's happening in my life. I think he'd be really proud of what I'm doing with my dogs and doing in his honour. Damn, here I go again, turning on the waterworks just typing this and thinking about him. Thankfully, I have my dogs right beside me to comfort me.

My dogs make me feel whole. As corny as this may sound, *they really do complete me.* They always have and they always will. It's who I am and I'm proud of it.

MY FIRST DOG: INTRODUCING SARGENT

Shortly after I was married the first time, my now-ex and I moved into our dilapidated house in Sebringville. I was taking a well-deserved break from renovations and sitting on the crooked, paint peeling front porch.

Ahh, the solitude of a beautiful sunny Sunday morning in a small village community. There really is nothing like it.

It was a particularly warm fall that year, and many of my neighbours were outside as well, but no one dared start up a lawn mower on a Sunday, not in this quaint little village. Relaxing in my lawn chair, sipping my coffee, and smiling to myself, I was in no hurry to get back inside to the job of painting the walls. Nope, no hurry at all. In fact, I was just going to close my eyes and enjoy the sun on my face. Absolute bliss.

THUD, BANG!

What the?! I jumped up. I thought the roof was falling down!

But what I saw was a huge black dog lying down next to me like he'd been there all along.

His gigantic tongue was lolling out the side of his mouth, and he was panting heavily. Pant pant pant.

I looked around. Surely his owner was around here somewhere?

"Hey buddy, where'd you come from?" I asked.

He had the sweetest eyes ever. Big, brown, soft, and extremely kind, and when I spoke to him, he scooted over a bit closer to me so I was within touching distance.

"Okay, I get it," I told him with a grin matching his. As soon as I started stroking his head, he leaned in further and that was it…we were pals.

He had a collar with tags. The tag read "Sarge" and had a phone number on the back.

"So, your name is Sarge, eh?" He looked at me dubiously, as though we were negotiating a deal. "You know I have to call your owner, eh Sarge? I would really love to keep you, but you do have a home and I'm sure they're missing you something awful because you're so darn cute."

At that point, Sarge put his head on my lap and I regretted ever looking at the darn tag.

I just couldn't stand the thought of some little girl or boy missing this amazing dog, though. I mean, if he was my dog and he had gone missing, I'd be absolutely frantic!

"Come on, buddy, we better go call your family." Ugh, I really didn't want to make that call. After I made the dreaded call, and left a message with our name and address on it so the owners could pick Sarge up, I thought the least I could do was play with him while he was still here.

Sarge and I had a great time! Even if it was short-lived. As soon as I heard my phone ring, I knew it would be his owners. My heart sank with every ring and I debated not answering, but I felt obligated.

A guy came to pick Sarge up, and I noticed that Sarge didn't run over to him like a lost dog who was happy to see his owner would. Hmm, red flag number one.

Then he told me that Sarge ran away all the time. Really? I thought. Red flag number two. Then I found out that he was a farmer and that Sarge was tied up outside to the barn and "somehow" kept getting off his chain. Red flag number three. And then came the big one…the farmer said, "It's getting to where he's not worth going after anymore! I'm thinking I'm just going to get rid of him." Bingo, red flag on fire!

"You don't want him?" I asked.

"Well, he obviously doesn't like it at our place," the farmer said.

Damn damn damn! I was recently married and knew that I had to start making these kind of decisions with my husband so I told the farmer that I'd talk it over with him when he got home from baseball and that maybe I would take Sarge.

"Well, let me know," he said. "You have my number."

That was the longest Sunday afternoon of my life! When my husband got home and I told him about Sarge, he was very skeptical. Whatever. I had done my duty as a wife and told him, so I called the farmer and got directions to his farm.

When I got there, I saw a very different, very depressed Sarge. He was chained to a steel shed.

I got out of my car, and when Sarge saw me, it was like seeing an old friend. He was so happy. I thanked the farmer, loaded up my new dog, and took him home. I had no idea that this dog would someday save a man's life.

Sarge was a cross between a black Lab and a Great Dane. He was around two years old when I got him and he only knew one command: "sit." I worked with him every day and he ended up being an extraordinary pet.

By the time I had a baby, I could say to Sarge, "Go get a diaper," and he'd run upstairs into the nursery and grab a diaper for me and bring it downstairs. I would heat up a bottle and leave it on the counter to cool and say to him, "Go get the bottle, Sarge," and he would run into the kitchen and grab it and bring it to me.

He could differentiate between toys, he would sing for me on command, he would, of course, bark or speak on command as well. He was so well-trained that he actually acted in the Stratford Festival Theatre's production of *Two Gentlemen of Verona*. If I couldn't take him myself, they had a special taxi to come pick him up.

He was truly amazing!

Now, obviously my marriage didn't work out, and sometimes when that happens people's lives get uprooted and that's what happened to us. However, I've always been a firm believer that everything happens for a reason. Sarge came into my life for a reason and now I had to find a new home for him.

I had just told my BFF Julie that I needed to find a home for Sarge when her eyes lit up. Her sister Jess worked at a pet store and just that day someone had come in looking for a dog for a man in a wheelchair! NO WAY, you say! Yes way, I say! Once again, fate had stepped in and everything was going to be okay.

Sarge and I went to meet Larry a couple days later. It was an instant connection. I saw how much Larry already began to love the dog that I loved in such a short period of time.

We worked together to train Sarge to help Larry in certain aspects of his life, especially when it came to Larry's emergency life line. It's something you hope you never need, but if you do, you want to make sure it's all in working order.

This is what we did. Sarge had always loved his "baby," a certain toy that he had. I brought it with me from my house. It had my smell on it, which was fine because this was not going to be his everyday toy; this was his emergency toy.

Next, we strapped "baby" to the emergency call button. This way, the minute Sarge grabbed that baby, no matter how hard, he would be making the call for help.

With the emergency operator on alert, we practiced. It didn't take long for Sarge to figure it out. Then, in hopes he'd never have to use it, the baby was put in a very special spot. A spot that Sarge knew of but was not to touch unless told too.

Saying goodbye to Sarge was probably one of the most difficult goodbyes I've ever had to say. Even though Larry encouraged me to visit, I knew it wasn't fair to either Sarge or him if I did. Sarge had to know that this was his home, and that he wasn't just visiting.

Larry and Sarge were the talk of Tavistock. They went everywhere together. Larry gave Sarge an amazing life.

Then came the call...from Larry.

It had been a regular day, he said, just like any other, when all of a sudden, he must not have paid attention to how close his wheelchair had gotten to the corner of the step and...oh my God, Larry said, before he knew it, he was hanging upside down, precariously dangling on his staircase.

I still get goosebumps when I think of that phone call. I could hear the fear in his voice.

What happened next was nothing short of incredible. Larry said Sarge was already there beside him, so he just said, "Go get your baby." And

Lucky's Way

just like that, Sarge took off and grabbed his baby, which signalled the emergency help call that ultimately saved Larry's life.

I was so unbelievably proud of Sarge. And so very thankful that he was there to help. Sarge was with Larry for around five years. Just an average dog who did above-average, extraordinary things.

Ironically, after my-now husband Bob and I met, I found out that he had bought the farm that Sarge originally came from.

I told him all about Sarge and Bob told me that after he bought the farm, the first thing he did was tear down the old barn and shed. He came across a five-foot chain attached to the corner of the steel shed. "I remember thinking, 'poor damn dog that was tied to this,'" Bob told me, saying that the chain was ridiculously short.

Continuing with the irony, the "farmer" who ended up giving Sarge to me actually got a job at the same place where I was working just before Bob and I got together.

He and his wife were very sweet people. I can't hold a grudge. Not against him. Some people just don't understand that a dog isn't an animal to be chained up to the side of a building and thrown food once a day.

Times have changed and thankfully, so have *most* peoples mentalities and attitudes towards animals. Over the years, our pets have become less looked upon like "just" a cat or dog etc, and more like a member of our family.

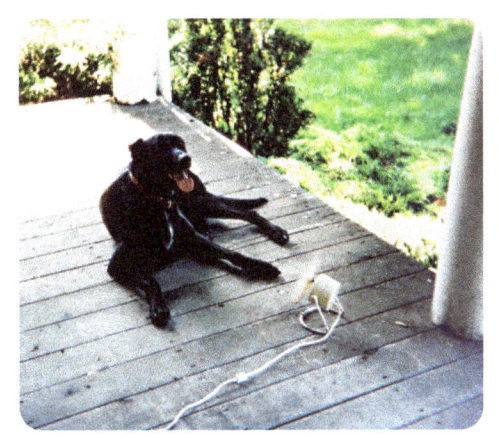

Sarge...the dog, the actor, the hero!

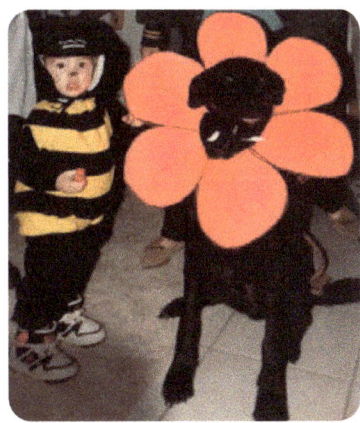

Spencer as a bee and Sarge as a flower.

CHAPTER 2

*My Therapy Dogs...and My Very Own A**hole Dog too!*

I want everyone to know, right from the get-go, that I'm not just writing a book about training dogs; I am living it as well. Yes, I too have an a**hole dog! Some people find that hard to believe because I'm a dog trainer.

Well, guess what, folks? It doesn't matter! My a**hole dog is my very own, very sweet Clark Griswald. He can be such a little poopster, I'm telling you! Hello, my name is Brenda and I own an a**hole dog.

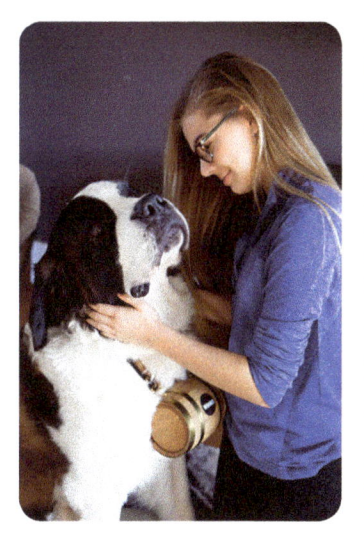

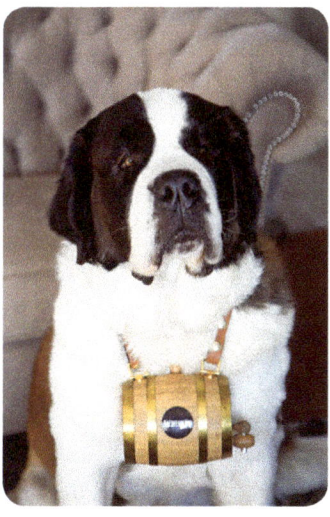

Clark Griswald, my very own a**hole dog...but he sure is good at acting cute–right, Brooklyn?

Brenda Boemer-Groenestege

MY FIRST THERAPY DOG: DOUG'S STORY

When I decided that I wanted to get a puppy to train as a therapy dog, I began looking into different breeds. A mastiff was my number one choice. An American mastiff, English mastiff, bullmastiff, or Neapolitan mastiff…it didn't matter; I just love the breed and wanted one. However, I called breeder after breeder and there were either no puppies available or a super long waiting list. Damn. I paid my fifty bucks and got my name on a waiting list and resigned myself to the fact that I would be waiting a while to get a puppy.

Fate, however, had a different plan for me. Thank Heaven!

It was Sunday night. We had just finished Sunday supper when our house phone rang. I picked up and was confused for a minute by what the lady on the phone was saying. Excusing myself to the office, I asked her to hold the line while I switched phones.

"Could you please repeat what you were saying?" I asked.

She laughed, and very graciously started the conversation again. "Hi, Brenda, my name is Laura and I got your name from our mutual vet. I had my Great Dane in there the other day for a checkup. I told her that my mastiff stud literally broke out the basement window to breed with my Dane and now we were about to welcome a litter of puppies from that mating! I also explained to Dr. Angela that because they were a crossbreed, I needed to find homes for them with people that I could trust. With people that I know will have them spayed or neutered when the time comes. Also, they need to be with someone that has prior knowledge of working with big-breed, strong dogs. And that's when she gave me your number. Are you by chance interested in a puppy?"

I couldn't believe my ears. "I'd love one of your puppies."

Laura went on to explain that they breed Great Danes and mastiffs, but not normally to each other, and therefore the puppies would only cost a portion of what I would pay for a purebred. Plus, she told me that I could have first pick when the pups arrived! Oh my goodness! I was so excited.

A few weeks later, Doug was born. He was so freaking adorable! I would visit him regularly a couple of times a week, so when it came time

Lucky's Way

to take him home, he was more than fine coming home with me. Training started immediately. He was amazing. A true natural.

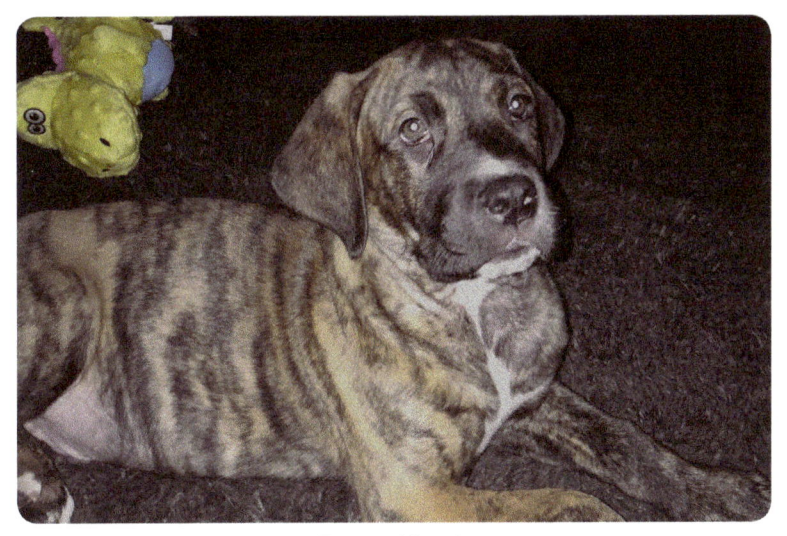

Doug at 10 weeks

I remember it vividly: it was a Sunday evening and I had received a call that one of my closest friends, Lizzy, had been taken to the hospital with stroke-like symptoms. I was shocked and scared. I told Lizzy's daughter that I'd be visiting the next day because I knew she had her entire family with her and didn't need any more excitement. Monday came and I loaded up Doug. It would be his first "official" day out as a therapy dog. I said to him, "Ready or not, we're going up to visit Lizzy and help make her feel better."

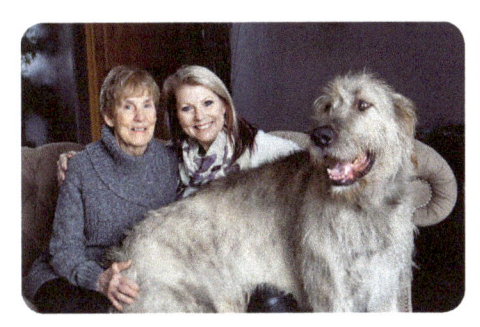

Lizzy, me, and Harold   *Clark Griswald, Lizzy, and me*

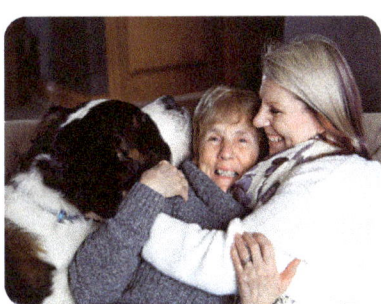

15

Off we went! Doug was seven months old at this point and we'd been training for this since the day I got him. I put on his therapy dog vest and we marched our way into the hospital to find our friend. Doug was already 115 pounds and quite tall, since he was half Great Dane and half mastiff, so he was an impressive sight walking into the hospital. He kept trying to pull me into certain patients' rooms, which confused me at the time, because he was usually so well-behaved and never pulled on his leash. I didn't realize that he knew instinctively which people needed him, and therefore I tightened my grip and essentially found myself needing to drag him along with me until we found Lizzy's room, which, of course, happened to be at the very end of the hall. Naturally, she was very excited to see us.

It wasn't long before one of the nurses came into Lizzy's room to ask us if we would be able to bring Doug into a couple of the other rooms to visit more patients. We were more than happy to do that. Doug already knew which patients needed him. Once the word got out that there was a therapy dog on the floor visiting patients, well, that was it…Doug was a very busy boy, making people extremely happy.

Doug dragged me into one of the rooms, where I noticed a gentleman lying on the bed. All of a sudden, Doug jumped on the bed with the man! I didn't know what to do! I watched as the man completely enveloped Doug in his arms and began crying.

At this point, a nurse walked in. I fumbled my words, trying to explain that I was so sorry about Doug being on the bed, when the nurse put her hand on my arm, and with tears in her eyes she said, "Oh my gosh, no, don't be sorry! He's been on suicide watch for days now because he's so depressed. He's been wanting to see his dogs but they're still back where he lived before, which is a twelve-hour drive away. This is amazing. This is just what he needed." Then the gentleman's brother came in and he was quite shocked as well to see a giant dog in bed with his brother, but again very happy at the same time.

When it was time to go to visit the next patient, I promised the gentleman and his brother that Doug and I would be back later in the week for another visit.

That was a promise I did not know I would not be able to keep.

In the room next door was a lady named Grace. The doctors and nurses explained to me that they weren't sure if she was "still in there" after her stroke. Grace would never acknowledge anyone, she would never make facial expressions of any sort: no smiles, no tears, no frowns…nothing. She wasn't making any sounds or noises. The only thing she would do was make the same back and forth motion with her hand, repeatedly. When we walked into her room and she saw Doug, her eyes lit up. I moved Doug over beside Grace, right under her hand, and then the motion she was making made sense.

Grace smiled! "Do you like that dog?" her roommate asked.

Grace nodded her head. When she did this, the doctors and nurses looked at each other and said, "She's there all right!" as tears streamed down everyone's faces.

"Would you like to see that dog again?" Dr. Mark asked, in his very sweet British accent. Grace nodded yes.

Again, I promised to bring him back to see her. Which was, once more, a promise that I would not be able to keep…damn, I hate not keeping my promises, but this was out of my hands.

The next morning, Doug was hit and killed instantly on the road. I was absolutely devastated. I got a call from my neighbour and very good friend Marg that her feed truck driver had hit him with his truck. I barely remember driving home from Stratford. Thankfully, it was only Bob who I cut off, almost getting into an accident. I didn't stop at the stop sign to turn onto our road, as I was racing home to find Doug's lifeless body in the ditch in front of our house and I quite literally almost took out Bob in his truck because he too had been called.

I had been grocery shopping with Judi, the school secretary at the primary public school where my daughter attended. We were picking up supplies for the grade eight graduation party that evening when I got the phone call. When I flew past Judi's car after getting the call from Marg, she knew something was very, very wrong and followed me.

It was Judi who pulled my sobbing, heartbroken body off Doug and walked me over to where Bob, Marg, and the gentleman who hit Doug were standing. Marg hugged me before I turned my attention to the feed truck driver.

He was very shaken up and felt terrible for hitting Doug. I gave him a hug and told him that I didn't hold him responsible. It was an accident.

After that, I excused myself, went into the house, and had a complete meltdown. Doug was everything to me. I spent every minute of every day with him. I took him everywhere with me and he was turning into an incredible therapy dog.

He had been so naturally intuitive, extraordinarily gentle, calm, loving…just an overall amazing dog. He brought so much joy to people, including myself, and I just couldn't imagine my life without him. I hugged his favourite stuffed toy and cried harder. Why? Why Doug?

What broke my heart even more was having to make the phone call to the hospital to let them know that we would not, in fact, be honouring our promise to come back. Having to explain what happened to Doug and cry, along with the nurse, was very difficult. The hospital staff was amazing and supportive.

I spent my days lying on the couch, crying on and off, depending on what commercial was on and if there was a dog in it. It was a very dark point in my life and there was nothing that anyone could do to make me feel better.

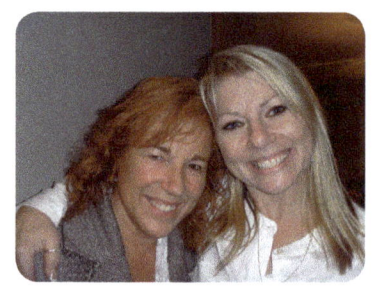

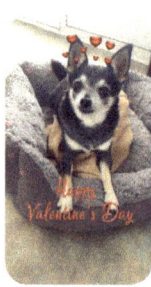

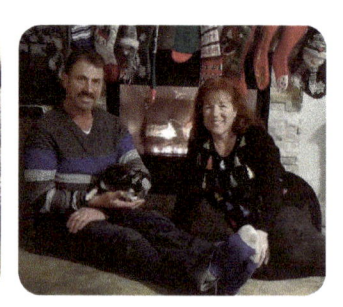

Marg and myself   *the Rudster*   *Pete, Marg, and Rudy*

Day after day, my friend Marg came over to check on me, knowing full well that I was very much *not* okay. She offered to bring her chihuahua, Rudy, over to comfort me, which always made me smile. Rudster, as we lovingly call him, is one of the only really small dogs that I have ever actually bonded with. Marg would sit with me as long as I needed her to. She would sit and listen while I ranted…why Doug? I just didn't understand! I was so angry with God. We were doing such good work and then, poof,

He took Doug away. Marg just hugged me, knowing exactly how I was feeling because she too has been through losing a fur baby on the road

One morning, very, very early in the morning, I had half woken up and I was still half dazed when I rolled over and went back to sleep. That's when I had a dream. A very, very vivid dream.

Any psychic or medium will tell you that when you dream about someone who has passed away, it means their soul is visiting you and you should pay attention to what they're saying or doing in the dream. In my dream, my dad said to me, "Doug vas just here to show you vat you ver going to do mit the dogs…now Harold, he's gonna take you all ze vay!"

I woke up immediately. The first thing I thought was, "What the hell kind of a name is Harold for a dog?" and then I laughed at myself. Laughed until I cried. The thought of getting another puppy, training him, loving him, and something possibly happening to him, was almost paralyzing to me. I didn't think I could do it. I just couldn't go through that again.

Later that day, my kids had popped over and Bob decided it was a good time to have a family talk. Which means he talks and everyone else has to listen.

He started off by saying that he knew it was really hard on me losing Doug. The day before the accident, I had had such an amazing day and I had come home so happy. He said that he wanted me to be happy like that again.

Bob continued, "You've been down and depressed for weeks and we hate seeing you like this. You're not cooking or baking, you don't laugh or smile, nothing. I can't believe I'm going to say this but you need to get another dog and start again. I don't care what kind you get, just get one and please get happy again!" He sounded so sincere.

I was already shaking my head no when my son Dylan spoke up. "Mom, you have to get another dog. You just have too. You started something really great with this therapy dog thing, so you can't just give up on it. You HAVE to keep going! I have a really good feeling about this, Mom. This is what you are suppose to do!"

I sat there for a minute saying nothing. I looked at my family. Spencer was nodding in agreement to what his brother had said (which was a miracle in and of itself…they never agree on anything). Bob and Brooklyn were just looking at me, waiting for an answer.

I told them about the dream with my dad. We all laughed and everyone agreed that yes, I did need another puppy, and his name would be Harold. Immediately after that, Bob said, "And just so you don't start to worry again, we're putting in invisible fencing for the dogs. We are not going through this again!"

I gave my husband the biggest hug I think I'd ever given him. "Thank you for everything," I said, meaning it from the bottom of my heart.

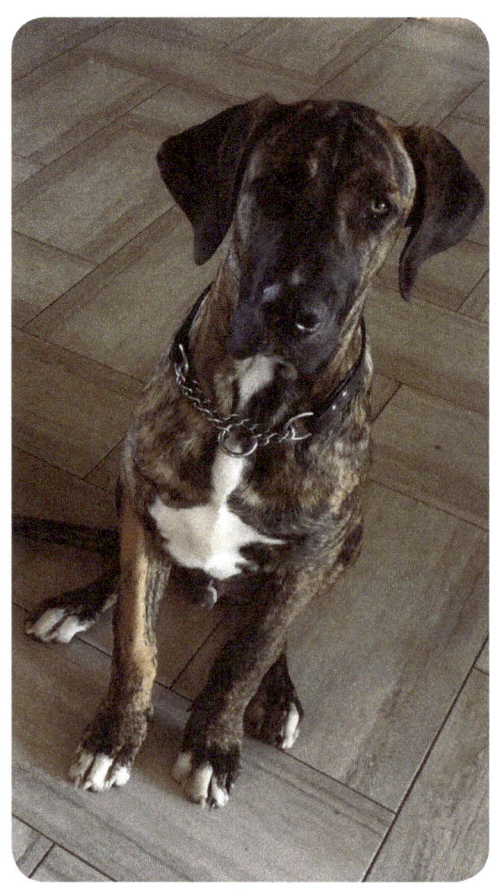

Doug…still missing you.

SERVICE DOG ORGANIZATIONS:
THIS MAY RUFFLE SOME FUR, BUT I HAVE TO SAY IT...

I might possibly upset some people or organizations here, but I think it is ludicrous that families in need of therapy dogs for their children are having to pay upwards of $25,000 for a dog. Again, this is *MY* opinion and I stand by it.

I was brought up with the understanding that you bring a puppy into your home at eight weeks old (approximately), and that puppy will bond with the child who needs him or her through sheer instinct alone.

Yes, of course there is training to be done with that dog to make it behave and become socialized properly, but again, with the right dog, that training can be done *by the family* with proper instruction from a professional trainer, without the price tag of thousands of dollars.

Now, don't get me wrong, *there are definitely exceptions here*! Seeing eye dogs, or service dogs of that nature, definitely need a higher level of training and are trained by professionals in that specific field.

I'm talking about autism, developmental deficits, PTSD, anxieties... these are the types of therapy dogs that, in my opinion, should be started with the child or adult as a puppy and worked with side by side with a trainer. And *NOT charged an arm and a leg for!*

It sickens me when I hear about families waiting years for a dog because they either can't afford one or the dogs are in such demand that there's a waiting list!

It's my full intention to start working side by side with families in need when my daughter goes off to university in a few years. I'm hoping to get as many dog breeders on board as possible to help me, by either donating a puppy or, at the very least, selling one at a lesser cost knowing that it's going to become a service dog for a child or adult in need.

Working with families and showing them how to train their own therapy dog can give them the tools they need to train their own puppy. When the time comes for another puppy, they will have the knowledge to train it themselves. *"Give a person a fish and they can eat for a day, but teach them how to fish and they can eat for a lifetime."*

How many times have you heard stories about the family dog that's alerted the parents because the child isn't breathing or is convulsing or something? Regular family pets do amazing things every day just out of sheer instinct, without any formal training.

I look at my own dogs as examples. They have their own personalities but, hands down, Harold is more in tune to people's needs than any of my other dogs and I've trained them all the same. If I'm not feeling well or am really upset, Harold comes into my room and literally lies on me. If I'm sobbing, he's in my face and won't leave me alone until he knows I'm okay. Why is that?

How does it happen that one dog is so much more sensitive to people's emotions or "vibes," for lack of a proper term? Why are some dogs more naturally instinctive or intuitive than others? Is it possible to train that into a dog? How do some dogs just know when you need them?

Case in point: One night my (unofficially adopted) daughter Victoria came over, kind of on a whim and kind of not. Now, she and her husband, Matt, have had some difficulties getting pregnant and were told that she was quite possibly never going to be able to get pregnant, no matter what means they tried, whether nature or science.

It was a devastating blow to them since they both adore children and wanted to fill their home with as many kids as possible, and quickly, after they got married. After mourning this soul-crushing news, they agreed to take a step back and not necessarily accept what the doctors and the universe handed them, but just to stop thinking about it, for the summer at least. They really needed some time to relax and enjoy each other and give themselves time to mentally, emotionally, and physically heal from this news.

Any couple who has gone through a similar situation knows how difficult this can be for relationships; even the strongest of couples can be torn apart when faced with fertility issues. Not only does it take an emotional and physical toll on the couple, but a huge financial one as well.

I was so proud of Victoria and Matt because of how strong they remained during this process. I sincerely think it brought them closer together rather than ripping them apart.

Victoria is an aesthetician, an amazing one, and the Monday before she came over, I had an appointment with her at the spa where she works.

I noticed she was particularly quiet. Normally we chat up a storm, about everything and nothing. But that day, she was just quiet…too quiet.

I wanted to ask her what was wrong, but deep down inside, I was pretty sure I already knew. It was the end of the summer and I was fairly certain that maybe her and Matt's marriage wasn't quite as resilient as I thought it was. So when she called me the next night and asked if she could come over, my heart sank. I thought I knew what was coming.

Victoria came in holding a gift bag. She was obviously carrying a bottle of some sort, and for privacy we went into my bedroom.

I smiled sheepishly and said to her, "So what's up, sweetie?"

"Here," she said, "this is for you." She handed me the gift bag, and I honestly thought, What the heck are you thinking, babe? You know I only drink Bud Light.

I pulled out a bottle of wine and at the same time I said, "You really didn't have to do this…" Then I read the label:

Only the best Parents get promoted to GRANDPARENTS
Baby Moore arriving April 2019

I looked at Victoria in absolute shock! I was literally stammering, "What? How? When?" and she was laughing and crying and simply said, "Just naturally." I grabbed her and started uncontrollably sobbing.

Harold came running into my room, jumped on the bed, and kept trying to get his head in between Victoria and I. He just wouldn't let up because I was such a mess. He kept pawing at me and laid himself across me as though he was afraid I was going somewhere.

It is a complete miracle for Victoria and Matt and I am the happiest soon-to-be Grandma or GG on earth! It took hours before the shock wore off that night and every time I thought about that wee miracle baby, I would start crying all over again and Harold would be all over me again. Gosh, it still brings me to tears just writing about it and, of course, Harold is right by my side comforting me.

Brenda Boemer-Groenestege

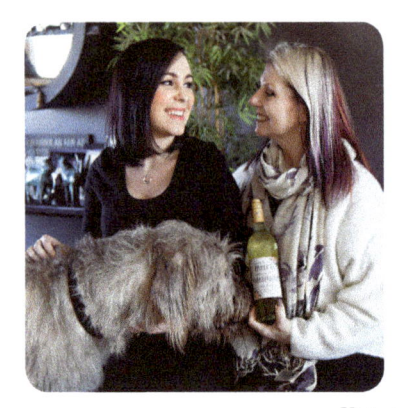

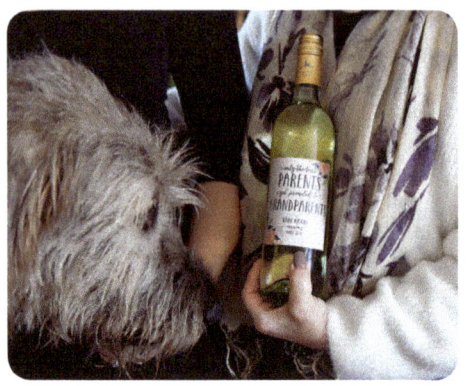

Victoria, Harold, and me

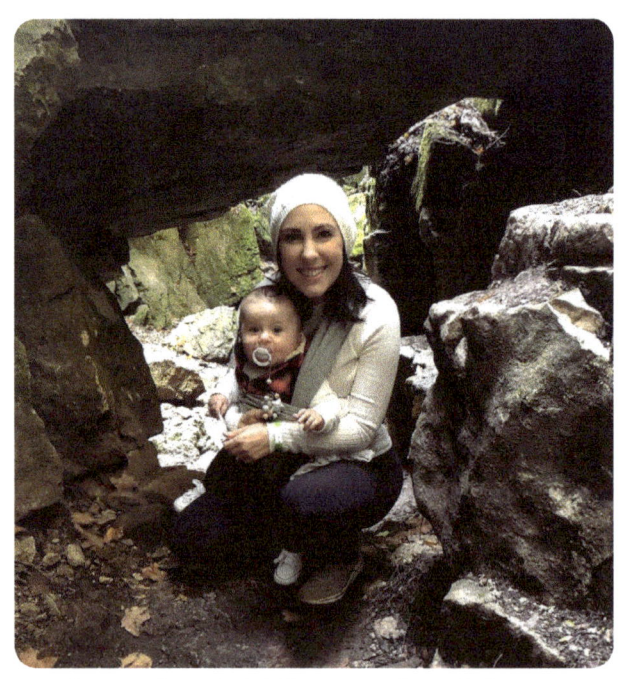

update: introducing Myles! He is amazing! Just like his mommy.

CHAPTER 3

The Bond Between Father and Daughter...and Dog

*The following chapter contains mature content and strong language and is not intended for young readers. Parental discretion is advised.

My father bought me my first German shepherd. He imported Irkos from Germany when he was nine months old. My ex, who I'll refer to as "he" (what? I could have called him much, much worse!), let's just say he wasn't the nicest guy behind closed doors, especially when you added alcohol.

I went to visit my dad on a beautiful Sunday morning. I had been telling Dad for months that "he" had been getting progressively more and more verbally abusive and his anger had begun scaring me, especially around my two very young boys.

Keep in mind that I was always a tomboy growing up, so normally my dad would just say something like, "You're a big girl, you can handle it," and brush it off, but that day, when I showed up to talk to him, it was different. Dad noticed something in me that I rarely show…it was fear.

I told my dad that the week before, I had come home unusually late from working overtime at my job with a local landscaping company. I had asked "his" parents if they could pick up our kids from the babysitter, since I would be working late, and stay with them until "he" got home from work, which was only a matter of an hour. Since his parents didn't work, I didn't think it would be a problem.

It had been a gruelling day. Twelve and a half hours of hard physical labour and I was truly exhausted. We had to get the job done since it was out of town, so we all pushed ourselves to our physical brink and every muscle in my body felt it by the end of the day.

Just keeping my eyes open driving home was a task in itself. I was dreaming of the nice hot bath I was going to take when I got home.

Pulling into my driveway, the first thing I noticed was that my in-laws' vehicle was still there. Damn. I just wanted to climb into the tub and then my bed. There was an anxious pit beginning to fester in my stomach. I knew this was not going to go smoothly.

When I walked into the house, "he" and his parents were sitting around the kitchen table drinking. Not a surprise. The question that came out of his mouth, however, did surprise me. "What's for dinner?" he asked, with a noticeable amount of sarcasm, since there was obviously no food in sight. I tried to keep my temper in check when I answered, "I just finished working over twelve hours; I'm pretty sure you can figure it out for once."

Yeah, that went over like a ton of the triple mix fertilizer I had shovelled so much of that day! I really didn't care. I continued walking through the kitchen, not breaking my stride as I headed to the stairs.

His face turned shades of red and purple and he flew out of his chair and screamed after me, "Are you f'ing kidding me? My parents did you a favour by picking up your f'ing boys and this is how you repay them? By being a total f'ing bitch! Get the f**k in here and make some supper!"

Now *that* stopped me in my tracks. I turned and looked at him. "I'm sorry, they did *me* a favour by picking up *MY* boys? Is that what you just said?" If words could hold fire, he would have been up in flames!

"Damn straight that's what I said! So the least you can do is make supper for them!" he spewed at me.

I knew my babysitter had, thankfully, already fed Spencer and Dylan, so at that point I decided there were just no words left to say to him...well, none that a lady should say anyhow.

I took one look at him and his parents, since they were now standing behind him nodding their heads in total agreement to what he was saying, and I turned my muscle-weary, dirt- and sweat-covered body around and continued walking through the living room and up the stairs, all the while listening to his ranting and raging. "You f'ing c**t (that was his favourite thing to call me—nice, eh?), get down here and make f'ing supper! Do you hear me, you f'ing c**t?" Oh, I heard him, I just chose to ignore him in favour of getting to my much-needed hot bath.

I could still hear them talking about me, so I decided to sit on the top step, lean my aching head on the bannister, and eavesdrop on the conversation between him and his mother while waiting for my desperately needed hot bath to fill. I heard something that truly shocked and disgusted me and justified what I needed to do next.

His mother—of all the people in the world, his own mother—said to him, quite matter-of-factly, "You know, honey, sometimes you just have to give 'em a smack or two to let them know who's boss." His father was in the background agreeing with her and making backhand sounds with his hands.

"She's gotta learn to listen to ya, sonny!" he said.

I was shocked. Were his own parents actually condoning abusing me? Who does that?

Then and there, I decided there was no hope in hell for my marriage if that was the kind of bullshit advice his own parents were giving him. I most certainly did not want my boys witnessing any of this and so the planning began. I had to get us away from him.

I decided I'd start by telling my dad. If you are a parent, you can imagine how unimpressed you would be, and my father was no different after hearing this first story. But then I had to tell him the rest of the story…and that was what happened on the following weekend.

I explained to Dad that he had come home after drinking with his friends at the beer tent after baseball. I still remember exactly what started the argument. One of his best friends, who suffers from "little man syndrome," decided, for some stupid reason, that he could prove to his buddies that he could do the "pile-driver" wrestling move on someone.

Well, of course, little big man couldn't pick on anyone bigger than him, so, completely unbeknownst to me, he walked up behind me (by the way, he was drinking too, shockingly) pulled me off my chair, and wham, flipped me over and did this crazy wrestling move on me that damn near broke my bloody neck!

I was in tears because it hurt so badly and I was also in absolute shock when I looked over at "him" to find out that he was not freaking out on his buddy for performing a wrestling move on me, his wife, that could have broken my neck! Nope, they all thought it was quite funny. I certainly didn't! Not then and not now! A**holes!

(Hey, maybe that should be the title of my next book…How to Remove All the A**Holes From Your Life, Past and Present; I like it!)

Anyway, I still have problems with my neck, thanks to that damn guy! I left "his" ass happily sitting in the beer tent and went home to my kids.

Of course we fought about it! He was pissed off at me for embarrassing him in front of his friends by leaving! Can you imagine that? I still shake my head at that one.

This time, though, I was not only really, really pissed off, but in pain as well, and I was not going to back down! (Now, in hindsight and therapy, I can admit that, on my end, I probably should have just kept my mouth shut and tried walking away…unfortunately, that just wasn't in me at the time.)

Spencer was already in bed and I was getting Dylan settled and ready for bed as well when he came home. For some reason, he wanted to take Dylan out of my arms. Now, any protective mother would do exactly what I did if their drunk-ass husband was trying to grab for their child. I told him no, he was beyond drunk, and then I tried to walk away with Dylan.

He kept after me. At first it was just a verbal assault, a litany of profanity that I won't even bother repeating. By that point, I really didn't care anymore, to tell you the truth. But then he started in with grabbing and "manhandling," for lack of a better term. Grabbing me, grabbing my clothes, grabbing anything. Anyone who's ever had their clothes pulled on hard enough knows that it can cause a multitude of injuries, including choking, from the tightening around the neckline, which then ends up leaving bruising. It can also cause a burning sensation, like a rug burn, and it leaves that kind of bruising rash (when the material is stretched to the point of ripping).

I still wouldn't give him the baby, who was now crying, as both of us were yelling (here's when I should have just walked away…again, 20/20 hindsight and therapy). That's when things got even more rough.

I did try walking away but he was adamant that he was taking Dylan! I tried to get past him and he got ahold of both of my arms and wouldn't let go. He was shaking me violently and screaming in my face and finally he shoved me against the wall! I hit my head hard. He knew he was hurting me but he was out of control!

After shoving me into the wall, he threw not only me, but because I was still holding Dylan, he threw *us* into the neighbouring chair. We landed hard but thankfully I could cradle Dylan to ensure his safety. I was seeing stars from when my head hit the wall, and I could feel blood trickle down the back of my head but I couldn't stop to help myself because his rant wasn't over yet. I was still holding onto Dylan with both arms and by this point I was seriously scared. I was screaming at him to stop.

Thankfully, Val, my neighbour, heard the fighting and came over. As soon as "he" saw her, he quickly changed his tune. There's something about witnesses that seems to make the behind-door-bullies change their tune. It didn't matter how nice he pretended to be; she knew what was going on and he knew he'd been caught.

And that brought me to my dad's.

The damage was bad. When I took my jacket off and showed my dad my arms, the look in his eyes was something I'd never seen. Then I took my scarf off and he saw the mark around my neck. He asked if there was any more. I pointed out the cut on the back of my head and the welt marks from where the clothes he ripped at had left their mark on my body. His face went from anger to absolute anguish and back. There were tears in his eyes that day and I knew they were from unbelievable anger. As a parent myself now, I can imagine what he must have felt.

He had to look away. When Dad looked back at me again, he said, very quietly, "I'll take care of it, Runt." I knew that he felt he had to do something. It's weird because I didn't go there in expectation of him "doing" something, I just went there because we had that kind of relationship. I didn't want my dad to fight my battles for me, and that's not what this was about. I just needed for him to know what was going on.

Dad said he would go and have a talk with "him." And by "talk," Dad meant threaten him, and I knew that would not go over well. "He" was always very remorseful the next morning, after he'd sobered up, and I knew that it would just make the next time worse if my dad went over and threatened him.

My father did what he thought was best; he took one more long last look at me and my damaged body and told me to leave it with him and I did. He was the one man I trusted.

A couple days later, I got a visit from my dad. He had called his contacts in Germany and ordered a protection dog for me. I cried tears of joy that day.

I was about to welcome what would become my protector, my hero…I hoped. He would not be just any dog, he would be a beautiful German shepherd.

My new dog came from a long line of professionally bred and trained protection animals. My dad's friend still breeds and trains German shepherds in Germany. He also still trains protection dogs for private citizens, as well as trains some dogs for Schutzhund, which includes obedience, protection, and tracking.

It was amazing to think that after thirty-plus years, my father still had these kind of connections to his past. Honestly, it made me really proud. More proud of him, I should say.

The day *finally* came when my German shepherd was flying in. I didn't sleep at all the night before because I was so unbelievably excited about getting him. Well, that and the fact that I also hadn't bothered telling "him" I was getting a protection dog. I mean, seriously, how do you think that would have gone over? How would I have even started that conversation with him?

"Oh, by the way, Dad bought me a German shepherd because you're such an a**hole and the next time you decide to manhandle me, you're going to have to go through my dog first! Hope you're okay with that." Nah, why bother, I like the surprise angle better.

My dad was adamant that no one but me was to handle my dog when he got off the plane in Canada. "Irkos Von Haus Licher" was his registered name. I was like a kid at Christmas the day I went to the Toronto airport with my dad's cousin, who we considered our uncle, Bernie, to pick him up.

I waited until all the passengers came through first. After what seemed like an eternity, and after watching package after oversized package being brought out, including other dogs and cats, they finally, finally brought out MY new dog.

As I crouched down low to peek into his crate, my eyes welled with tears. I knew he was feeling overwhelmed with everything going on. I could only imagine that he would be leery of me, but when our eyes met, there was something in them that told me I could trust him. And I hoped he saw the same in mine.

He was beautiful. Absolutely gorgeous. It was truly love at first sight, at least for me. Oh Lord, I wanted to take him out immediately and just run my hands around his head and neck, hug him and kiss him and reassure him that everything would be all right and that I'd take care of him and love him always.

I was desperate to get him out of that damn kennel and love on him like only a crazy dog mom can with a new puppy, but alas, I was reminded that it wasn't permitted inside the airport. Dog kennel in tow, I walked as quickly as my twenty-eight-inch legs could walk to get him outside so I could properly pull him out and have a good long look at him.

He really was a magnificent-looking animal. He was long and lean, sleek, very dark in colour, and had eyes that only the person he loved could really trust.

All the way home, I stroked his head and comforted him until finally we arrived at Uncle Bernie's house. After reloading in my vehicle, we headed straight to my parents to show my dad what his investment looked like.

When we got there, my dad looked Irkos over and approved of him wholeheartedly. He said to me, "Hang on to him, Runt. Hang on to him good," and before I knew what he was going to do next, my dad hauled off and punched me right in the shoulder!

Holy balls did that hurt! But more importantly, my new dog reacted immediately and lunged at my Dad, missing his skin by mere millimetres! Irkos almost ripped his sleeve off!

I have to admit, I was so caught off guard I almost tinkled myself when it happened, but I was also secretly, incredibly thrilled with what I had just witnessed! More importantly, my dad was extremely impressed by Irkos, and, thankfully, not hurt.

He repeatedly said, "That's a good dog!" Unfortunately for my dad, after that day every time he came near me when Irkos was with me, my dog would go after him. And I mean go after him. I guess it really is true what they say…you only get one chance to make a good first impression!

As far as my ex is concerned, we all know there are two sides to every story, right? Well, this is my side of the story…

It was the night my Oma (Grandma) Boemer flew in from Germany. I had gone to the airport with my dad to pick her up and by the time I got home, it was later than I had anticipated.

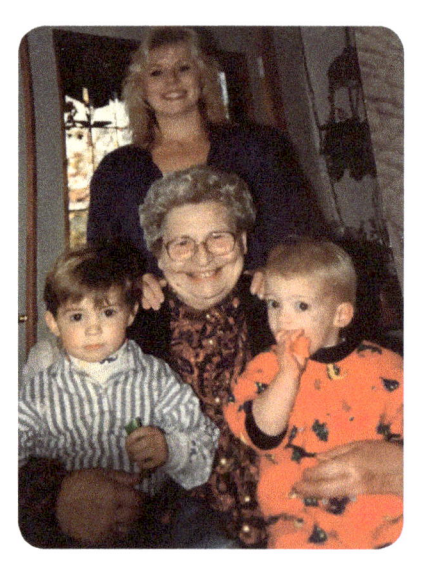

My Oma Boemer with Spencer, Dylan, and me, the day she flew to Canada

It never went over well if I didn't have dinner ready for him when he came home from work, let alone if I hadn't been home when he got home. He had been drinking, which was par for the course, but as always, that escalated his anger.

I had put Spencer to bed (he was two and a half years old at this point), and Dylan was crying because he was hungry and tired, and needed a bottle and his bed. "He" followed me upstairs, yelling at me and berating me about being a shitty f'ing wife, and how it's my duty to have his dinner on the table because he worked hard all day and blah, blah, blah.

I told him I really didn't care and that he was a big boy and could make his own damn dinner. Now, by this point, his head was pretty much turning purple and about to blow off because he was so angry. It didn't matter to him that I had gone to pick up my grandmother from the airport.

Irkos was between us the entire time, which just elevated his anger even more. He had hated my dog since the day I brought him home. It had been bliss for me, though. Even at night, Irkos would sleep right beside me and make sure that he didn't come over to my side of the bed, if you know what I mean. If he tried something, I would pretend to be sleeping and Irkos would be draped over me, growling. Anyhow, back to that night.

I still had Dylan in my arms when all hell broke loose. "He" snapped. He tried to grab Dylan out of my arms and I spewed a litany of obscenities at him. I called him every rotten name in the book! I had had my fill. I was sick of him. I was tired, had a migraine, and the last thing I needed was this overgrown ass having a bloody temper tantrum because I wasn't home to cook dinner! Give me a break already!

"You're a grown man! You can start making your own damn meals! And if you don't like it then you can move back in with your f'ing mother because you two deserve each other!"

He swung. I put my hand up to block the blow, so he connected with my thumb instead of my face. It hurt something awful, but it was him who was screaming bloody murder, not me. It took me a second to realize what had happened. I was thinking, Why the hell are you screaming when you punched me…but then I realized that Irkos had got him and I ran.

I took off with Dylan and ran into Spencer's bedroom. I sat on Spencer's bed and held Dylan on my lap. Irkos ran in and jumped up onto the bed. "He" was hot on our heels.

He grabbed me around the throat and was threatening to punch me but Irkos positioned himself between me and him. I had one arm around Dylan and one hand holding Irkos back from attacking him.

He was screaming, "Your f**king dog bit me! Do you hear me, you stupid f**king c**t? I'm going to kill that dog!"

I said, "Either you let go of me or I let go of him! Your choice!"

He opted to let me go. Wise choice, I'd say.

Yes, Irkos had bitten him, but only because he was protecting me and Dylan. I was so proud of Irkos that night.

I ended up with a broken thumb, which now, twenty-five years later, I've had to have surgery on because of the arthritis brought on by the original break, but I'm thinking it could have been so much worse.

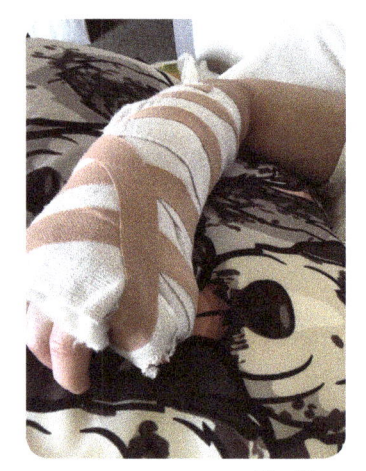

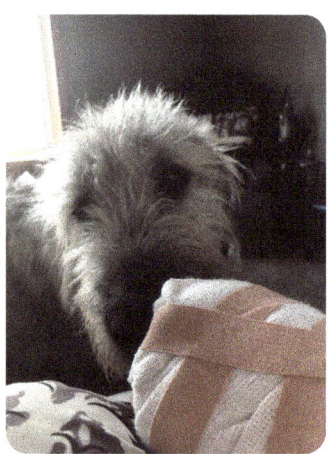

Harold never left my side.

Irkos and I had a very strong bond, and he definitely stopped the abuse that was going on inside my house, which ultimately ended in a divorce.

For about a year my boys and I had to move into Stratford into a townhouse. I couldn't take my dogs with me, so Irkos was living at my parents', outside in a big dog kennel. (This was when Sarge went to live with Larry).

One day, my dad asked my mom, "What's wrong with the Runt?"

My mom replied, "Nothing that I know of, why?" Dad pointed outside to Irkos's kennel. He was going absolutely bananas! He was jumping from side to side, making the kennel rock like crazy!

Dad told mom to call me. He said "Something's wrong with the Runt and he knows it." Sure enough, when my mom called I was in the midst of a really bad migraine and I needed a ride to the hospital. I had been just about to call her. (At the time, we lived approximately six miles apart.)

So, how did Irkos know? Is it possible for a dog to know their owner is in trouble from so far away? Could it really be possible that he knew

Lucky's Way

I was in pain from so far away and in need of help? Makes you wonder, doesn't it?

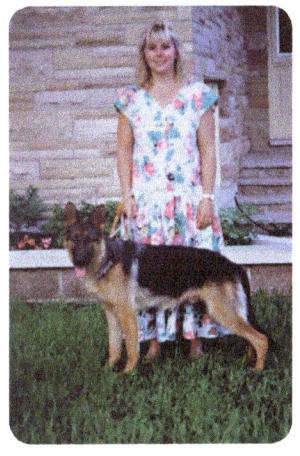

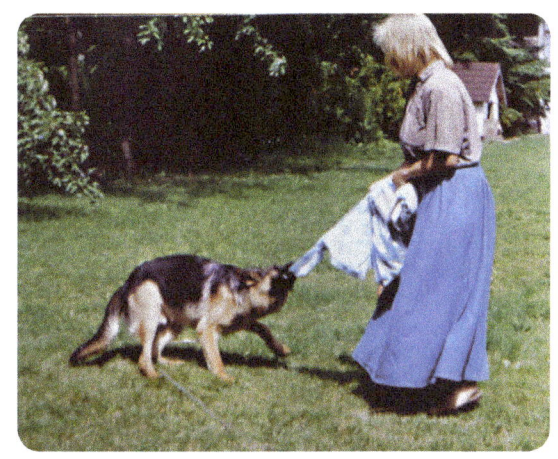

The day I got Irkos

Training with Irkos

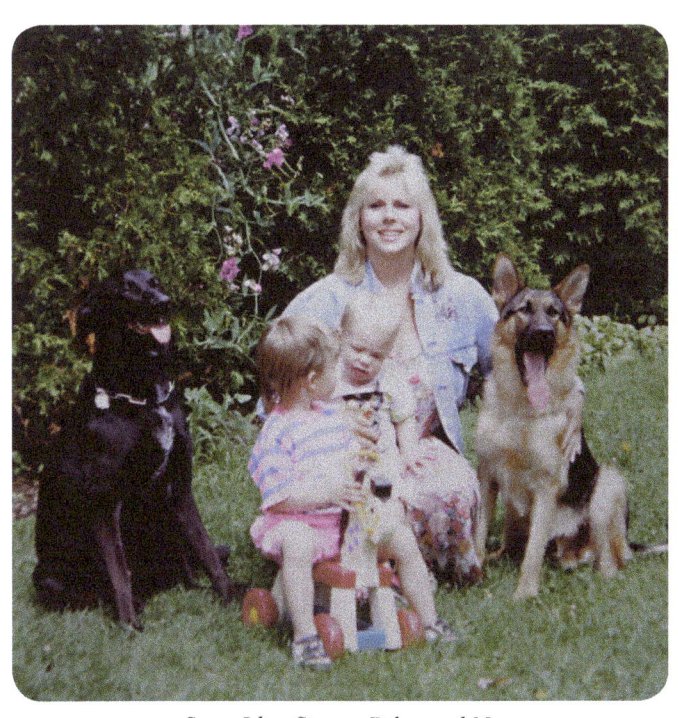

Sarge, Irkos, Spencer, Dylan, and Me

I decided to tell my story because it showed not only the bond I had with my dog, but also the bond I had with my father. This is, unfortunately, how my life was, and how a lot of other peoples' lives have been, and still are. If you are suffering at the hands of an abuser, please contact your local women's shelter or police department, and tell a friend or a family member. You don't have to go through this alone.

–Brenda

CHAPTER 4

The Bonds We Make

When I am down with one of my migraines, I can always count on Harold to be by my side, if not Lloyd and Leonard as well, all comforting me, lying next to me in bed. Just having them with me while I'm feeling like crap definitely helps ease the pain a bit.

While writing this book, I had a back spasm that damn near sent me to the hospital. I couldn't believe the pain I was in! And it came on so fast; I was turning around to grab some spices while I was baking and BAM, it started to seize up. I started repeating, "No, no, no, no!" and my husband looked at me and said, "What the hell are you talking about?"

"My back! It's cramping up! Oh shita, shita, shita!" I whined back at him. He looked at me like I had three heads, and asked the obvious question, "Why? What did you do?" Frustrated, I glared at Bob, because this has been a recurring issue with my back, and spat through clenched teeth, "I'm pretty sure it's from having to pick up my a**hole dog Clark to get him in the truck when it's time to leave therapy and go home!"

At this point, I gimped my way to my bedroom, grabbed my heating pad along with a couple of painkillers, and headed over to my easy-boy chair. After a little while sitting in my chair and drinking tea, I had to use the washroom, and getting from a sitting position to a standing position was NOT going to happen! I couldn't stand up for all the money in the world. The pain running down my lower back was something I've never felt before (and I've delivered babies!).

I called out Harold's name and, of course, he came right over. I gave him the command to "stand firm" and he did. I used him to help push myself up. He helped me walk to the bathroom, stood in front of the toilet until I was finished, and helped me up again, and, well, you get the picture, right? For three days straight, until I could see my massage therapist and chiropractor, Harold was my saviour. I walked on a forty-five-degree angle, in absolute agony, and Harold stayed with me night and day. He really is my hero.

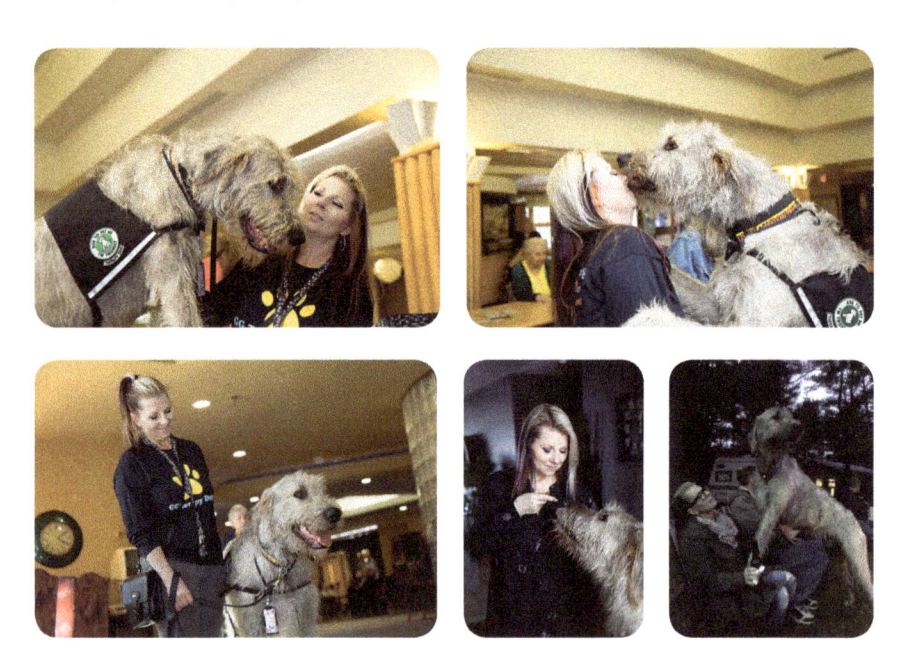

IS IT REALLY POSSIBLE TO HAVE A BOND THAT STRONG WITH YOUR DOG?

It was my father's belief that a dog bonds best with a person (adult, child, whomever) right from the minute he or she brings that puppy home at eight or nine weeks old. Perhaps even younger, if you're lucky enough to live close by where your breeder lives and can spend time with the puppy in the weeks prior to bringing him or her home.

Don't get me wrong; dogs have the ability to bond with people at any and all ages. However, in my father's opinion, when training a dog for a specific job (i.e., service dog, protection dog, police dog…etc.), the younger the pup, the stronger the bond. Again, this was his opinion, but who am I to argue? His methods have been proven to work time and time again and that's made a believer out of me.

TRUMAN AND EARL…THEIR AMAZING RESCUE STORY

Brooklyn and her friend Lana were an adventurous pair of eight-year-old girls when they decided they wanted to follow my husband behind our house to the edge of our property and go into the bush.

This is not your average backyard bush, by the way, it has acres of dense trees and brush, along with considerable foliage. There are also a couple of small streams that run through it and after a good rainstorm they can collect quite a lot of water before slowly turning into generous pools of mud. It was absolute heaven for a couple of imaginative girls on the hunt for a bit of exploratory adventure!

Bob went back to the bush to clear some brush and cut down some of the trees that had fallen in a storm. He was also cleaning up the riding paths to make sure they were all safe for the kids and adults who ride through the bush on four-wheelers and dirt bikes.

I told the girls to take along our dogs at the time: Truman, our big Saint Bernard, and Earl, our harlequin Great Dane. Brooklyn was also to bring her cell phone and her boat whistle with her, but, shockingly, the two giggling girls not listening to what Mom said and excited about going on an adventure together forgot to take the cell phone and the boat whistle.

Thankfully, they did take along their trusted hounds, or rather deck crew (they were big into *Pirates of the Caribbean* that summer). First Mate Truman and Buccaneer Earl ran off after "Captain Jack," aka Brooklyn, and "Joshamee Gibbs," aka Lana, as they went down the path to the wide open sea or, as we call it, our bush, to begin their great adventure.

Our bush is a good kilometre behind our house, and it was quite some time later that I got one of my mom feelings that something was not quite right. You know, that tingling feeling at the base of your neck that makes you stop whatever you're doing and check on your kids?

I stuck my head outside our back door and noticed that it was quiet… too quiet. I called to the girls. Hmm, no answer. I gave a whistle…still nothing? Huh, weird. Then something else came to my attention. My mom radar started pinging high alert because I no longer heard Bob's chainsaw either.

I didn't want to panic because I could hear Bob's voice in my head saying, "Oh my God! Seriously? You are always thinking the worst! We were just checking things out in the bush and you panic! I'm surprised you didn't call the bloody police department and report your kids were missing!"

I forced myself to remain calm. I refused to give in to the urge to panic. Besides, I was in the middle of baking muffins. What would Martha Stewart do? I thought to myself. So, channelling my inner Martha, I stayed focused on getting the muffins finished and out of the oven before I decided to panic about the kids.

As it happened, I had just pulled the muffins out of the oven and was looking out the window when I saw Truman running around the side of our barn. Whew, I thought, they're on their way back. Thank you, Martha, for keeping me focused.

I went outside and realized it was only Truman, and I immediately got a bad feeling, thinking it was really odd because normally Earl beats him home every time. And when I say normally, I mean *every single time* and by a long shot Earl beats him home.

Crap! Crap! Crap! Panic! Panic! Panic! My mom radar was spiking at nine out of ten!

I started the water running into Truman's bucket and he didn't want it. Okay, now that was *the* absolute very last straw! Mom radar is now at fifteen out of ten!

Truman started making this marbling sound. It's a sound that he made when he was *really* trying to get our attention. Like, when he was seriously wanting you to focus on only him.

Sometimes he would stand directly in front of you, staring right in your face, and make that sound non-stop until you would get up and either let him outside or get him a drink of water, or the best was when he would walk us over to the refrigerator and stand directly in front of the freezer and do a little prance and this marbling sound so you'd get him some ice cream. (Not just any ice cream; it had to be Haagen-Dazs because he loved Haagen-Dazs Half the Fat vanilla ice cream. He had standards.)

Lucky's Way

So I knew when he came home and made that marbling sound, something was going on and I needed to pay attention to him. I said, "Where are they, Truman?" He ran toward the barn, or so I thought, but when I headed in that direction, he started barking at me and ran over to where our gator (a four-wheel-drive, side-by-side ATV) was parked on the opposite side of the house. Holy crap, he's telling me to get on the gator, I thought.

As soon as I headed for the gator, he starting running toward the bush, and I followed him in hot pursuit.

It felt like an eternity before I got to the entrance of the bush. When I did, I turned off the engine and hollered as loud as I could possibly could, "BROOKLYN! GIRLS!" and whistled over and over. Please God, I prayed, let me find those girls! Then I held my breath and waited for a response.

Truman came up behind me, panting so loudly I couldn't hear anything except him. "Hush, Trum," I snapped, "I need to listen for them." As though he knew what I was saying, he walked over to a little puddle of watery mud, lay down in it, and was very quiet.

I hollered again and strained to hear anything from the girls. Finally, I heard them! Very, very faintly I could hear them yelling back for help. I had to close my eyes to determine which direction they had yelled from. I was pretty sure I had it, so off we went, Truman and I, and that's when it dawned on me…Bob was nowhere in sight!

Heading in what I hoped was the right direction, I continued to scan the bush for any signs of the girls. I repeated the process of turning off the gator's engine and hollering for the girls until I finally reached the point where I was confident that I could find them on foot. The girls had strayed from the groomed paths, which was a huge mistake, even for feisty pirates.

The bush gets so dense during the summer, and the girls had no idea what side of the bush they were on after they found themselves turned around a few times. Then, when they finally did manage to find their way out of the bush, they came face to face with a fully mature field of corn stalks!

That's when the girls got really freaked out. When I finally found them, they were both crying. Since they had wandered off the path, they had some fairly nasty cuts and scrapes from the dense weeds and tangled thicket. They were thirsty and they were definitely scared, but at least they had had Earl and Truman with them.

When I asked Brooklyn what happened, she explained that they got turned around in the bush and then they simply got distracted following their imaginations and before they realized it, she didn't recognize where she was. She said she knew enough to search out the "light," thinking that that would automatically bring them right back out onto the path to go home, but obviously it just brought them out of the bush and up next to the corn field, and she knew they were in trouble.

She said that they started screaming for her dad, but they didn't hear him anymore, so she did the only thing she could think of…she told Truman to go get help. Brooklyn said she grabbed his face with her hands and looked him right in the eyes and said, "Go get help, Truman! Go get Mom!" and he took off through the corn field. Earl stayed with them, never leaving their side. In the bush are raccoons, deer, coyotes, skunks, and we've even spotted wolves, so the girls had good reason to be scared, but they were well protected with Earl by their side.

Boy, were the three of them happy to see me! And I was happy to find them all together and in one piece.

After I got them home and cleaned up, Bob came home. I relayed the story to him and he was absolutely shocked! He had had no idea the girls had even followed him out there in the first place, and when he had gotten a flat tire and left the bush hours earlier to get it fixed, he didn't give a second thought to letting me know he had taken off, let alone left the girls behind.

So, what's the moral of the story? Average dogs do above average, amazing things out of sheer instinct.

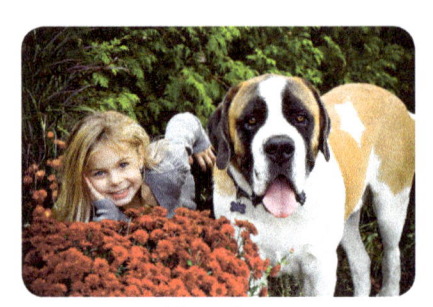

Brooklyn and Truman

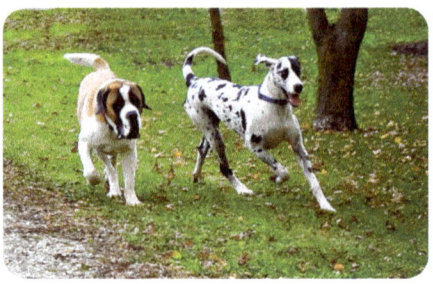

Truman and Earl

CHAPTER 5

Making the Right Choices

Finally, let's get down to picking that puppy! It's always such an exciting time when you and your family decide to get a new puppy. If you're looking for a dog to do a specific job, then *do your homework*.

Regardless of colour, gender, age, religion, political beliefs, disability, etc., all dogs ever really need from us is the basic necessities of life: food, water, shelter, and love, but responsible dog ownership has us now asking a few more in-depth questions:.

- *Do I/we have time for a dog?*
- *How do we introduce a new dog or puppy to our existing pet?*
- *Purebred? Mixed breed? Shelter dog? What's right for you?*
- *What size of dog?*
- *Do we need a hypoallergenic dog?*
- *Is dog hair an issue? Are you a neat freak, in other words?*
- *Do you plan on using this dog as a service dog? Will my child need the dog to go to school with them? Or does the dog need to go to my job with me?*
- *What's in our monthly budget to maintain a dog?*
- *Will we be traveling with our dog?*
- *Should we get a male or female?*

It can be quite the journey when it comes to finding your dog/puppy. Emotionally, of course, but physically as well. Depending on what breed you are looking to get, or what dog you are looking to adopt, you may find yourself driving, or even flying, to go pick up the newest member of your family.

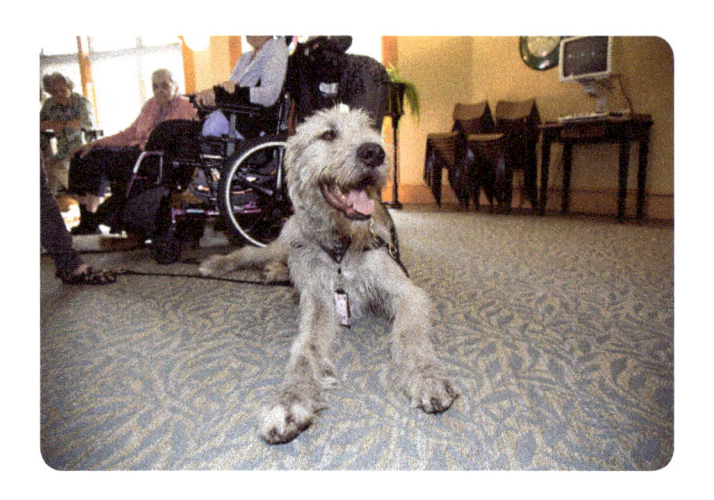

Answers to the Questions:

DO WE HAVE TIME FOR A DOG?

If your dog is going to be at home alone, in a crate or even just on its own for longer than six hours a day, I would re-examine whether this is the right time for you to get a dog at all. Dogs are pack animals and can suffer if left on their own for longer than six hours at a time.

Now, that being said, there are plenty of ways to get around this issue if you really want a dog but you work long hours. You can hire someone to come in and dog sit and there are always professional dog walkers available. A friend of mine adopted a dog from a shelter, and after he introduced his new fur family member, Buddy, to his neighbours, they began to offer to take him for walks while he was at work. It's an ideal situation if you have retired neighbours who enjoy dogs but don't want the full-time responsibility of dog ownership. This is really something to look into. It benefits all parties involved.

There's also doggy day care, for people with busy lives. This way, your dog has fun and becomes well-socialized with other dogs, and by the time you pick your sweet angel up, your puppy is happy to see you and it's dinner, maybe a quick walk, cuddles, and bedtime.

Quite often people make the mistake of thinking they should get two dogs so their dog will have a playmate. It is true that your dog will love the company of another dog, but keep in mind that two dogs, left alone for long periods of time, can also do twice the amount of damage in your home while you're away.

INTRODUCING A NEW DOG OR PUPPY TO YOUR EXISTING PET

It is very important to make sure that your current pet or pets at home are open to a new family member prior to actually committing to a new dog or puppy. If you have a well-socialized dog, then chances are he or she will be just fine when you bring home a new family member. That being said, always keep a close eye on them and watch for signs of aggression from either dog.

In the case of adoption, it's always good to bring your current dog with you when you go to visit the shelter or foster home where your future dog is living. Watching how they interact there will give you a good indication of how they will get along at home.

It is always a bit more challenging to introduce a puppy to a cat, depending on the personality and temperament of the cat. Usually, if the cat isn't impressed by the newest addition, they tend to ignore it as long as possible and then tolerate it when all else fails. In the case of adoption, make sure you ask repeatedly if the dog you are looking to adopt is cat-friendly. Otherwise, you may have a war on your hands when you bring your new baby home.

PUREBRED? MIXED BREED? SHELTER DOG? WHAT'S RIGHT FOR YOU?

Hands down, my all-time favourite all-around breed is the American Mastiff. Sounds funny, right, considering I don't actually own one myself? However, my son Spencer has one and she's absolutely amazing. Her name is Hemi and she has been a dream dog. She's very good with children, very patient, very calm, yet protective when the need arises.

Usually people have an idea of what they are looking for, so it's just a matter of doing your homework and finding out as much as you possibly can about that dog so you go into owning it with your eyes wide open.

One thing that you must remember is that dogs have been on this earth for thousands of years and they have deep-rooted instincts—instincts that don't go away just because the dog becomes your little angel.

A hound of any kind will always be a hound until the day they cross that damn rainbow bridge. Whether it's a beagle, who'll follow their nose until they can't physically run anymore, because they've collapsed due to absolute exhaustion or…their little legs fell off, whichever happens first, or a sight hound like an Irish Wolfhound, who will attempt to go through a plate glass window because of a reflection of a squirrel running up a tree (true story: Harold almost knocked himself unconscious at Greenwood Nursing Home trying to catch that darn reflection squirrel, and every time we go there he still looks for it to seek his revenge), a hound is a hound is a hound, and will always fall back on its basic and most natural instincts when push comes to shove, no matter how much you dress them up in little costumes.

I realize that most people will choose a dog almost the same way they choose a mate…by sheer attraction. My father always told me you can tell the personality of a person by the kind of dog they own. I wonder what that says about me. I guess I have a giant personality? Anyway, when you are choosing a breed, of course you're going to be attracted by its appearance, but please, please do some homework on it as well.

A herding dog will always have the need to herd. And it is a *need*. It's their most *basic instinct*. It's amazing to watch when trained and performed properly, but it can also be very scary to watch a dog attempting to herd a group of kids who have no idea what the dog is doing and are screaming in terror. Now, that's not saying just because you don't own sheep you shouldn't own a herding dog. There are plenty of ways to work around their need to herd. Quite often, depending on where you live, you can find local "herding groups" where you can bring your dog and hone its skills, if that's what you're interested in.

Lucky's Way

Keep in mind that every breed has specific characteristics. So crossbreeds, or designer dogs, as some people like to call them, may have multiple character traits and ingrained instincts in them that go back thousands of years! Wow, now there's something to think about. So, hypothetically, if some mad crazy breeder bred a beagle to an Irish Wolfhound, does that mean they would potentially get a dog who would run into a plate glass window at a reflection squirrel repeatedly until his poor little legs fell off?

At the end of the day, the more homework you do about the breed of dog you're wanting, the better off you and your future dog will be. Depending on what city and what country you live in, there are also professionals who will help you search out the perfect breed and then help you find your forever dog…for a fee, of course.

However, if you really have not given what breed you are interested in much thought, then maybe adopting from a shelter is an option. This way, quite often you get a dog that is already partially or even fully trained, depending on the circumstances of its history. Going to your local shelter can help you narrow down your search for what breed you want or, at the very least, give you an idea of what breed you don't want.

If you decide to get a dog from a shelter, please, please, please, take your dog to the vet within the first forty-eight hours and get it looked over! I've heard and seen too many stories of people adopting a dog from a shelter like the Humane Society, and then two weeks after bringing it home, the dog suddenly presents with some issue or another and after a vet visit, it's discovered that there is a huge problem with the dog that was there all along. Most shelters, including the Humane Society, don't have the funds to do extensive testing on all the animals that come in. Therefore they are unaware of the deeper issues with them and after forty-eight hours you have no basis on which to return the dog or get any financial help from the shelter and it will end up costing you big time.

That doesn't mean you shouldn't look into rescuing a shelter dog, that just means before you commit to the dog, bring it to your vet and have it checked over really well. You wouldn't buy a used car without having your mechanic look at it, would you?

> *If you adopt a dog or puppy from a shelter, get them checked over first or within the first forty-eight hours of ownership!*

If you have chosen adoption, I want to give you a couple of things to keep in mind for when you are physically at the shelter. I realize that every shelter dog has a sad story of some sort but I would like you to please try to focus not on the sad history of the dog but on the dog itself when you are moving from kennel to kennel.

Eye contact: if you are looking to adopt a power breed, for example, a German shepherd, Rottweiler, Doberman, pit-bull, Saint Bernard (I could go on but you know what I'm getting at), or a combination (mixed breed) of any of these breeds, I want you to pick up on whether or not the dog will make direct eye contact with you. If so, do they glare at you, even for a split second, before turning away? Or do they have soft, loving eyes and make a connection, even quickly, before turning away?

Dogs communicate using their eyes, among other things, but in this instance, when you're looking at what's quite possibly a dog with a questionable history, along with the fact that you are also looking at multiple dogs, in that split second of eye contact, that dog is telling you to either back off or that he/she is ready to be loved.

A dominant dog will control a situation using "hard staring" or "glaring" looks, and I'm sorry to say that unless you are highly qualified to deal with aggressive types of behaviours, I'm going to ask you to trust me when I say to pass on that dog and continue on until you find the right one for your family. We caught Harold using his dominant glare on Leonard by sheer coincidence while taking pictures for this book (you can find those pictures on page 114).

Please understand that I'm not implying that power breeds should not be adopted; I'm simply saying that unless you know and have experience with these types of dogs, they may not be a good fit for a first-time dog owner or for a family with young children.

I completely believe that you will know instinctively the dog that you are suppose to adopt almost immediately. You will feel it in your gut, and when you bring that dog home from a shelter, you will not be sorry.

Dogs are very forgiving and love goes a long way when it comes to adopting a shelter dog. They are normally so grateful and happy that you brought them home that they end up being the best dogs ever.

When people ask for my advice in regards to whether or not they should get a puppy or a rescue dog, fifty percent of the time I refer them to dog adoption programs or shelters because adopting a dog suits their lifestyle better than starting from puppyhood.

DO YOU NEED OR WANT A HYPOALLERGENIC DOG?

The meaning of "hypoallergenic"; hypoallergenic pets still produce allergens, however, because of their coat type, absence of fur, or absence of a gene that produces a certain protein, they typically produce fewer allergens than others of the same species. People with severe allergies and asthma may still be affected by a hypoallergenic pet.

If you're looking for a hypoallergenic dog, there are actually quite a few breeds to choose from and now, thanks to designer dogs, there are even quite a number of crossbreeds that are considered hypoallergenic.

When I asked the question about hair being an issue I'm speaking from experience. Saint Bernards *shed like crazy* (and let's not leave out the lovely drool), so if you're a clean freak, I would not recommend a Saint Bernard! Other dogs that shed include Labs (certain seasons are definitely worse than others, but they shed all year round, I'm afraid), Golden Retrievers, Newfoundlands, German shepherds…the list is long. Regular grooming can make shedding more manageable.

There are also the short-haired breeds like boxers, mastiffs, Great Danes, beagles—again, the list is long. With short hair you may not have to worry about the lovely "dog hair tumbleweeds" that roll gracefully around your house on a daily basis, but you'll still be sweeping regularly. Short haired dogs have their own set of challenges, if dog hair bothers you, for example, the short hair tends to stick to people's furniture and clothing in a way that long hair doesn't, and in cold weather months, short haired dogs quite often require a sweater or jacket to help keep them retain their warmth.

Again, doing your homework before purchasing a dog will help you in the long run by cutting down on your future house-cleaning services.

If you are not certain whether you or someone in your family is allergic to dogs, ask your family doctor. They can arrange an allergy screen, which will tell you whether or not you will be able to move forward with any and all dogs or whether you should be looking strictly for hypoallergenic breeds.

Hypoallergenic dogs are great for people with allergies because they either shed very little or not at all, making people less likely to have reactions to them.

Here's where the clarification comes…there is really no such thing as a *completely* hypoallergenic dog! Yes, unfortunately that's the ugly truth—the saliva and the skin of a dog can still trigger an allergic reaction in very sensitive allergy sufferers.

If you are an allergy sufferer, please check with your doctor before getting a dog or puppy. Doing this beforehand could ultimately save a lot of anguish and grief. There's nothing worse than bringing a new puppy home and having your family fall in love with it only to find out that you are still having allergic reactions and, in the end, having to give away your new pet. It's heartbreaking and could have been easily avoided. Your doctor should be able to give you a definitive answer as to whether or not you will be able to tolerate a dog.

Some hypoallergenic dog breeds:

Airedale Terrier
Basenji
Bedlington Terrier
Bergamasco
Bichon Frise
Border Terrier
Bouvier des Flandres
Cairn Terrier
Chinese Crested
Giant Schnauzer
Havanese
Irish Water Spaniel
Kerry Blue Terrier
Labradoodle
Lowchen
Maltese

Miniature Schnauzer
Poodle (Standard, Toy)
Portuguese Water Dog
Puli
Shih Tzu
Soft-Coated Wheaten Terrier
Standard Schnauzer
Tibetan Terrier
West Highland White Terrier
Wire Fox Terrier
Wirehaired Vizsla
Xoloitzcuintli
Yorkshire Terrier

Again, I can't stress enough, do your homework before buying or adopting a dog. Get all the information you can find and educate yourself before making such a life-altering commitment.

DO YOU PLAN ON USING THIS DOG AS A SERVICE DOG FOR YOU OR YOUR CHILD?

If this dog needs to accompany your child to school, or if you need to take it with you to work, you may want to avoid some of the giant breeds like the Irish Wolfhound, the Saint Bernard, or the Old English Mastiff. For one, they take up an enormous amount of space, and two, the drooling breeds… well, they drool, which in and of itself can be very unappealing to some.

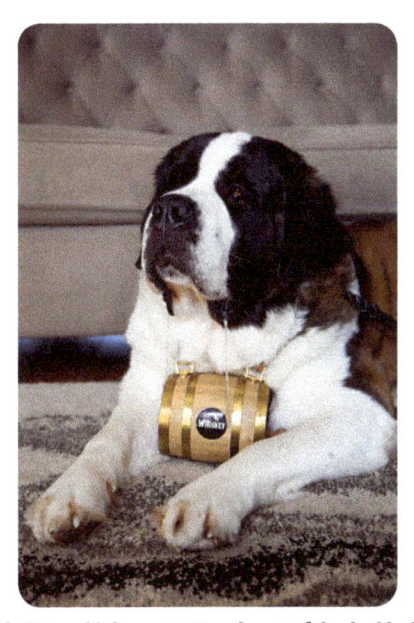

Clark Griswald demonstrating the art of the double drool.

If this is the case, there are still many, many dogs you can choose from. Please don't ever rule out a mixed breed dog either. For one, they tend to be healthier because they don't seem to have the sort of generational physical or mental issues that come with certain breed bloodlines, and two, they *should be* a heck of a lot cheaper!

When I say *should be*, I mean it! Don't get sucked into paying through the nose for a "designer" dog. You are actually paying for a mutt.

Sorry, kinda got off track there, but as far as service dogs go, there's nothing wrong with a mutt/designer dog for a service dog. It's all in the training. Just make sure you know what you're looking for when you go to pick one out. Again, this may be a good time to ask for help from someone who knows what characteristics to look for. Believe it or not, you can spot them from a very early age. That's where having faith in your breeder, if you can't be right there, is key. Explaining that you are looking for a dog to train to be a service dog for your child or yourself/partner is a key piece of information for your breeder.

When I go to pick out a puppy, one characteristic I look for is whether or not I can lay the puppy on his back, and if he will let me tickle his belly. This is one way of showing that I will have a calm, even-tempered dog.

Another trick I like to do when I go to look at a puppy is to call all the puppies over, then, when they are all running toward you, clap your hands really loud or make another loud noise and see which of the puppies didn't shy away. Pick the puppy that didn't shy away. That puppy is already showing more confidence and that is what you are looking for in a puppy. You want a confident dog, regardless of whether or not you will be training it for therapy. A timid dog can be very difficult to socialize and therefore train.

One more thing to watch for when you go to pick your puppy: don't get so distracted by the cuteness of the puppies that you don't pay any attention to the mother dog. A friendly, confident, social mother dog is a sign of good, positive nurturing for puppies. If the mother dog is anxious, nervous, or timid, these are traits that you want to pay special attention to. If the puppies are exhibiting the same type of anxiety, I would reconsider taking this puppy home. I encourage you to get to know your breeder early on, and if at all possible, go there and visit the puppies so you can see for yourself how the mother is behaving.

Having the luxury to visit your puppy prior to the day when he or she becomes officially yours, will also help to alleviate separation anxiety when it comes time to take your little pup home because he or she already knows and trusts you. I like to bring a blanket from my house and give it to the puppy while he is still with the mom. This way, my smell is already beginning to imprint on him and he bonds faster.

WHAT IS YOUR MONTHLY BUDGET TO MAINTAIN A DOG?

After you and your family have decided on the breed of dog, then comes the budget. First things first: the actual cost of a specific breed of dog is hard to determine until you do your homework. You shouldn't have to take out a second mortgage to buy a dog.

When it comes to budgeting for dog food, ask your breeder how much food the adult dog eats in a day. And *please please please,* people, I love my dogs more than air, but buy the dog food that you can AFFORD to feed it! Don't go broke trying to feed your dog better than you or your kids eat! At the end of the day, you still need to live, right?

Here is a basic guide to give you an idea of how much dog food could cost you in a month.

Large Breed Adult Dog Food - NOW Fresh 12lb bag$55.99

Grain-Free Small Breed Adult - NOW Fresh 12lb bag $56.99

This amount will last you approximately two weeks for a large breed dog and a month for a small breed dog. For the giant breeds, it will last for less than that. Most dog foods also come in larger sizes.

Next, call your local vet clinic and find out how much it is going to cost to get all the upcoming vaccines as well as the cost for spay or neutering. General annual vaccines are likely to cost you in the neighbourhood of three hundred to five hundred dollars per year, depending on the size of your dog, and this includes flea and tick prevention as well as the worm medication that dogs need to stay healthy. This all goes together with responsible pet ownership. This is always a good time to decide whether or not you should buy pet insurance for your dog. It can save you hundreds, if not thousands, of dollars in the long run.

Now comes the part of the budget that people tend to blow crazy amounts of money on…toys, treats, and costumes! It's incredible how much money it takes to keep Fido looking spiffy, right? How many frilly dresses does Buttercup need? Ten? Twenty? And don't get me started on Halloween! Look, I'm as guilty as the next crazy dog person when it comes to dressing my poor dogs up and embarrassing the hell out of them in the name of doggy designers gone wild, but don't break the bank is all I'm saying.

KEEP IT WITHIN YOUR BUDGET

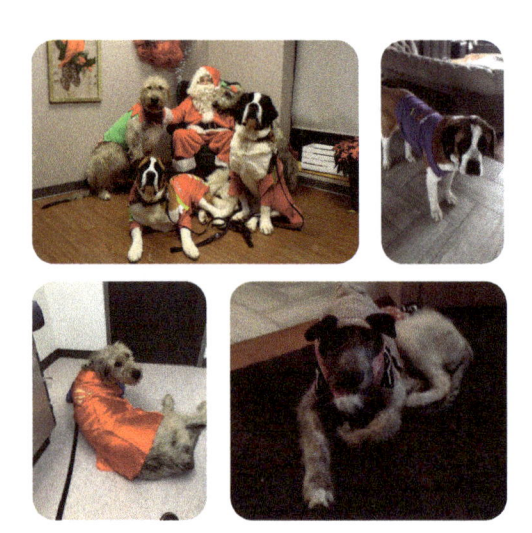

TRAVELLING WITH YOUR DOG
Something To Consider When Picking A Puppy?
Will you be traveling with the dog? In a vehicle, an RV, or maybe even on an airplane? There are things that you must take into consideration if you are wanting or needing to take your dog across the border or on an airplane.

If you are crossing the border with your dog, you must show up-to-date vaccine certificates signed by your veterinarian. I also choose to travel with a copy of anything else pertinent to my dogs: for example, a copy of their training certificates, their pet insurance, their registration papers, their microchip and/or tattoo information, a signed letter from your veterinarian with a picture and detailed description, etc. Anything that might come in useful in an emergency situation or in case your pet gets lost or stolen and you need proof of ownership.

In the case of flying with your pet, you will need to contact your airline provider in advance to determine whether or not your dog can ride with you or whether they have to be put in a crate under the airplane. In either case, there will be a charge for this.

If you have a service dog and you need them to travel with you, then you must provide proper paperwork from a doctor or psychologist/psychiatrist explaining that this is a service dog and that it must remain with you at all times. You will be required to pay for a seat for your pet. Likewise, to bring your therapy dog on the airplane with you, you will need a letter from your psychiatrist or psychologist stating that your dog is an "emotional support dog" and, depending on the size of the dog, you may have to pay for a seat for him/her. Again, you must contact the airline ahead of your flight to prepare them for your service dog or your emotional support dog to be on board.

Any time you are travelling with your pet, it is wise to ask your veterinarian if you should medicate your dog (or cat, for that matter) for the duration of the flight or road trip. It is not uncommon for animals to get motion sickness.

If you are taking your pet on a long flight and there will be no way for them to use the bathroom, my advice is to withhold food and water on the day of travel. During your travelling day, allow your dog very small amounts of water so they do not dehydrate, but wait until they have arrived at their final destination before allowing them to have as much food and water as they desire.

If you're a family who flies often and your new dog needs to fly with you, again, maybe an Irish Wolfhound or any of the giant breeds wouldn't be the best suited unless, of course, money is no object and they could fly first class with you.

If you are taking a road trip with your pets, it's very important to allow your dogs to get out and relieve themselves regularly. I would still follow the same rule as outlined above, however, since vehicles tend to be more constricted, unless you are in an RV. It's not only better for your pets to stretch their legs, but for you as well.

When I went to pick up Leonard, my younger Irish Wolfhound, my breeder asked if I would bring home a puppy for a couple in Stratford who had just purchased one from another litter but couldn't make the drive. When the owners came to pick up their new Irish Wolfhound, Wilbur, they were driving a two-seater convertible sports car. Yup, we teased them! Mind you, Wilbur looked smashing in the passenger seat of that sports car! We travel with our dogs in our RV. It's the best way to travel with a family and dogs, in my opinion. Although you have to be careful. Leonard decided, when he was six months old, that he wanted to be a dashboard dog *while* Bob was driving! Picture that, a hundred-pound Wolfhound puppy climbing onto the dash! We didn't know if we should laugh or freak out, so Bob did a bit of both before I got him down.

One VIP! *(very important point)*

One more very important point, while we're still on the subject of family dogs. I can't stress this enough.

Please do not buy your child/children/grandchildren, etc. a dog as a gift, or tell them that the dog is "their dog."

Dog ownership is a huge responsibility and unless your child/children are at an age where they are mentally, emotionally, and physically able and *wanting* to be responsible for the care of the new dog, you may just find yourself taking care of that dog all by yourself anyway!

Dr. Phil likes to say that "past history is a good indicator of present and future behaviour," meaning if your kids had a goldfish and never took care of it after having it for a week…you get my point, right?

The novelty of that new sweet little puppy will, unfortunately, wear off sooner rather than later, especially when it comes to doing the chores for the dog, and when it does, you will end up being the one taking care of them. So, unless you and your spouse/partner want a dog, *DON'T* get one.

The other problem comes at the end of the dog's life. What if something awful happens, like an accident, or the dog gets really sick and a decision has to be made to either spend an arm and a leg on the dog or put the dog down and all of a sudden your kid pipes up and says, "NO, you can't, it's MY dog!" Well, now you've gotten yourself into a huge predicament. At the very least, keep it as a family dog and divide the duties up according to keenness. And make sure that everyone knows that the adults have the final word.

In our house, they are my dogs and I do everything for them…but it is pretty darn handy living with a teenager who needs money and therefore will pick up poop for cash!

While on the subject of giving a puppy to someone as a gift, or surprising that certain someone with a new puppy… I would *not* recommend it! Definitely not unless it's something that the person in question had previously expressed interest in. This sounds very hypocritical coming from me because I have quite literally shown up and handed my husband a puppy before but, and that's a very, very large BUT, it almost backfired on me the last time! Let me tell you what happened…

I hadn't realized how badly Bob was missing having our big Saint Bernard Truman around. It was late Spring, and as a farmer, that's the time of year that you are always outside and your dog is *always* right there next to you. That spring though proved to be a very difficult one for Truman and unfortunately, we did have to say goodbye to him.

I didn't realize how much Bob missed having a dog that followed him around until I heard him trying to call Lloyd, Harold or even Leonard, who was just a very young puppy at the time, to come outside with him. It broke my heart to watch because he'd call them and they wouldn't budge from my side… they were and are very much *my* dogs, and my shadows. I can't describe the feeling that I felt when I watched Bob close the door and walk outside alone. I'd quickly give my dogs the command to get outside, now that Bob was out of earshot, and tell them to go get daddy. I'm pretty sure Bob knew that I kicked them out, but none the less, he was happy for their company.

Keep in mind that I'm already feeling extremely fragile because I know how badly Bob was missing Truman, before I tell you what happened next… again, fate or coincidence, whichever, I never miss a sign from the doggy spirits… I open my phone and what do I see? Puppy Saint Bernards! Come On!! It was a message from Lloyd's breeder. One of Lloyd's sister's had babies. Darn cute babies!!

And then it starts… it's like an addiction. I start making mistakes… it all starts innocent enough;

Mistake number 1 - I asked Lloyd's breeder if they are all spoken for? Unsure, she gave me the phone number of the puppies breeder! That was *mistake number two*! Because then I had to know right? It was just a question so I sent off a quick text to the breeder and asked… *mistake number three*! Damn it!!! Not only did she tell me that they were all still technically available, but then she sent pictures of the previous litter's so I could see what they would potentially look like all grown up, along with pictures of the dad and, of course, all the pictures of the puppies!!! *Mistake number four* is coming up super quickly now… "how much are you asking for the puppies?" I texted, secretly hoping that they were going to be ridiculously expensive so I could easily and conscience free say, 'no thanks, good luck' and go on with my life… but you **know** that's not how the story goes right?

While this was all going on, I'd been in the process of packing up our RV because we were heading out on a camping trip. Brooklyn was helping as well. Here's where I make the biggest of the mistakes of all… I showed Brooklyn the pictures of the puppies! *Mistake number five!* There was no going back then, I don't think I can even count that high I was making so many mistakes!

One thing was for sure, there was no mistaking that we could NOT let Bob know that we were even considering another dog. We already had three, and that was three too many in Bob's eyes, so this absolutely had to stay a secret!! No-one can find out! And for seven weeks we kept that secret to ourselves, all the while planning on how we were going to surprise Bob with his new puppy.

Here's how it all went down; I asked if I could pick up Clark Griswald on Sunday morning because Bob & the kids went golfing. We had ordered a whiskey barrel with Clark's name on it and put it, along with a cute Chevy Chase's Christmas Vacation Clark Griswald t-shirt and the puppy, of course, into a big box. When Bob came home, we sat him down and gave him his gift. He said right away without even opening it, "whatever it is, I don't want it", Brooklyn and I were jumping out of our skin in anticipation and Bob was being, well, he was being Bob!! So frustrating!!! "Just open it Dad!" Brooklyn said.

When he did finally open the top and saw something move, he damn near hit the ceiling! "what the f-bomb is it?" He yelled as he jumped out of his chair! Thankfully, Brook and I were close enough to catch the box so it didn't fall. We laughed as we pulled out Clark and we introduced Bob to his new little buddy, thinking he was going to love him. Ummm, yeah, that was not the reaction we got! He was furious! And I mean **furious**!!!

"Take it back! I mean it! Take the f'in thing back right now! We do not need another f'ing dog! What the hell were you even thinking? Why would you think this was a good idea? I'm serious, take it back, I don't want it!" He ranted on for a good ten minutes. "Why would you not have asked me first about getting another dog?" He questioned.

"Seriously Bob? If I were to have asked, what would you have said?" I knew this was a rhetorical question but I asked anyway.

"I'd have said hell no! We do not need another f'ing dog Brenda!" Bob answered the way I knew he would.

"Exactly, Bob. I knew you'd say no and that's why I didn't bother asking. I got Clark for you. Whenever you go outside, take him with you. Wherever you go, take him along. You need another buddy Bob." I said emphatically.

"I don't want one. We don't need another dog. Take it back. I'm not going to like it, I don't care! Get rid of it!" But by now the bluster had already gone out of his voice.

"Look, from here on in, I *promise* no more surprise puppies okay?" I said as sweet as I could be.

"I want that in writing," he said, "signed in blood!"

Ten minutes later, I'm watching Bob with Clark Griswald. Bob's reclining in his chair and Clark is laying on him. "I don't even like you you know? Go lay on the road!" He's saying to Clark. "You're not cute at all. Look at the size of your head for God sakes! People are going to make fun of you!"

The rest, as we say, is history. Clark Griswald is very much Bob's little buddy. He adores his daddy and vice versa.

I don't think I'll ever surprise Bob with another puppy again…

One last thought here: if you are the person who is the main dog lover in the family, which I happen to be in mine, then please make sure that you have made plans for what would happen if something happened to you. Who will take care of your beloved pet? In my house, my Irish Wolfhounds, Harold and Leonard, would go to my son Dylan, because he has such a strong connection with Harold, and, well, Leonard and Harold are a package deal. My husband, Bob, has an obvious soft spot for our Saint Bernards, so I'm not too worried about them, but I definitely needed to make sure I had a plan, or a *"will,"* for the others.

Something to think about, right? Also, if you are going to leave your pet(s) to a loved one, make sure to allocate a certain amount of money in your *will* to help take care of them, since the annual costs can add up.

Okay, Okay…that was two thoughts!

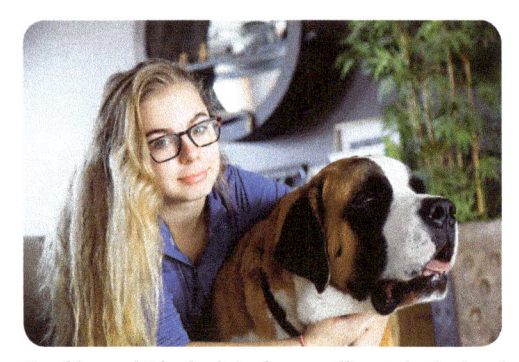

Brooklyn and Lloyd…she's always willing to lend a hand

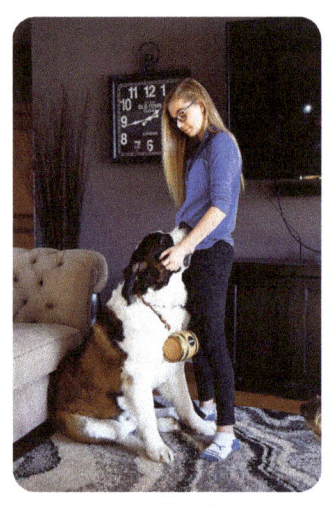

Clark Griswald and Brooklyn

MATCHING YOU WITH THE PERFECT DOG PARTNER - MALE OR FEMALE?

Here is the rule of thumb as taught by my dad: if you are looking for a family pet, I would recommend a female dog, because of their loving, nurturing nature.

If you are looking for a guard dog, look into a male dog. I'm not saying that females can't be, or wouldn't be, good guard dogs, but in my experience male dogs tend to make better guard dogs.

Lucky's Way

If you are looking for a dog for a specific child, for example, if you're wanting a service dog for your autistic son, then buy him a female dog, or if you want a service dog for your special-needs daughter, then I recommend that you buy her a male dog. This is something my father taught me years ago; he said that they would always match up females or bitches (if we are using correct terminology) to male police officers. The same rule applies if you're looking to buy a dog for yourself, hence the reason why I personally have four male dogs.

The reasoning behind my father's theory of matching male with female was really quite simple... hormones! He explained to me that by strictly using the laws of nature, animals are automatically drawn to the opposite sex; much like how they find a mate. Okay, so now you've decided which gender you want. Now you have to decide what breed is right for your needs, then find a reputable breeder, or perhaps adopt a dog from a shelter or an adoption group. Either way, it's time to do more research and get as much information as possible. Remember, owning a dog is a commitment and not a spur-of-the-moment idea. Again, *do your homework*! When it comes to getting a dog, you do not want to have buyer's remorse after the fact!

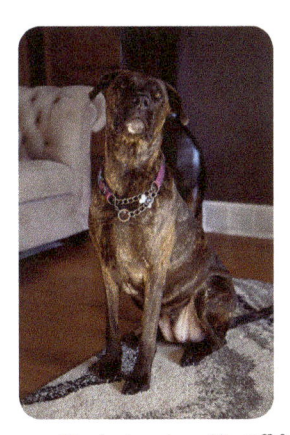

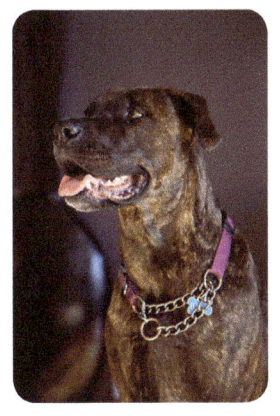

Hemi...American Mastiff female (my son Spencer's dog)

MY ROAD TO FINDING HAROLD

First I'll share my own story about how I found Harold. After getting the lecture from my family about needing to get another puppy to be a therapy dog, I began thinking about what kind of dog I wanted. Then it hit me! Bob had said he didn't care what kind of puppy I got as long as I got one, right? Well, that was my ticket to get the dog of my dreams! An Irish Wolfhound! Julie, my BFF, and I always said we wanted to get a pair. She would get a female and I would get a male. I called her immediately and told her what was going on, to see if she was ready for her Wolfhound puppy. Unfortunately, Julie and Joe still had their little dog Reggie at that point, and they both worked full-time jobs, so it wasn't the right time for a puppy. I completely respected their choice.

My reason for choosing the Irish Wolfhound breed is multifaceted. I had a friend years ago, who had one and he was absolutely gorgeous. His name was Cedric. He was a big, loving teddy bear and I fell in love with him. Irish Wolfhounds are very calm by nature, which is perfect for what I had planned for him. I've always been drawn to giant breed dogs. The bigger the breed, the more laid back they seem to be.

My search for Harold began. I started calling around to multiple breeders in and outside of Ontario before I found the breeder that I felt I connected with the best.

Before I tell you about her, I have to tell you about one of the funnier, and crazier, breeders I had to deal with. It still makes me laugh when I think about it.

She was in the States. Ohio, to be exact. She wanted to come to our house for a four-to-six-day time period (she would decide when she was here how long she would be staying, whether it would be four or six days) to assess our living situation before she would approve us as "adoptive parents" to one of her puppies. Thankfully, we weren't on FaceTime or she would have seen the expression of complete "You must be crazy," on my face! She continued to say that she would be flying in…at my expense, of course, and she had some very strict dietary concerns that she would email me. "Umm, okay…" I said, and she continued on that she must have a window seat in the airplane *and* on the drive in the vehicle to and from the airport she insisted that she must sit in the front passenger seat because she gets motion sickness in the back seat.

I was trying really hard not to laugh in her ear over the phone when I asked her if there was anything else that she would *require* while she was here (it took every ounce of my being not to call her "your highness"!). Hold onto your hats, everyone, it gets better: the bedding must be one hundred percent cotton, and it would need to be freshly laundered every day! She also asked for a bottle of Perrier water, unflavoured, at her bedside every evening before she retired for the night. You can't make this stuff up! Lastly, upon her leaving, *if* she approved our home for one of her dogs, we must give her an eighty percent down payment for the puppy (in cash) to hold him for the adoption.

Now, considering the cost of these particular puppies was more than the down payment on my first home, and the fact that I found this woman completely obnoxious, I felt the need to explain to her that, number one, I wouldn't be adopting a puppy, I would be purchasing one. I'm not sure why that term rubbed me the wrong way, but it did. Number two, there was no way in hell that I would spend that kind of money on a puppy coming from her! The price easily doubled because of her thinking she's some kind of celebrity big shot who's going to be flown in and treated like royalty under the pretence of assessing my house for a puppy! That dog would have cost me well over ten grand!

"Well! I'm totally offended!" was the last thing she said to me before I hung up the phone, laughing my head off.

I made a few calls to other breeders before I found *my* breeder, Julie Beamish, who owns Norhunter Irish Wolfhounds. As soon as Julie and I started talking, I knew she was the right breeder for me. (I know this may get confusing since my BFF's name is also Julie, so I will use "BFF Julie" whenever I'm referring to her, so everyone can differentiate between my BFF Julie and my Irish Wolfhound breeder Julie.)

I told Julie that I was looking for a male puppy and that I would be training him to be a therapy dog. I told her about Doug, and we both cried on the phone together, knowing the pain of losing a loved pet. I explained to Julie that I needed a puppy who was calm and chill, and I really wanted a big male with a boxy square head. She understood immediately what I was looking for, and told me about a litter that she had. The puppies would be ready to go home on August 12. I smiled and took that as a sign; that was my dad's birthday.

Now, since Julie lives in Sault Saint Marie, which is an eleven-hour drive from me, I obviously couldn't just jump in my vehicle and drive up there to see the puppies myself, to verify that she was a legitimate breeder. So, how do you verify your breeder under these circumstances? Julie has a Norhunter Facebook page that she added me to, so I was able to see and talk to all the people who had previously gotten puppies from her, along with people who were waiting on puppies from the same litter as me. Very exciting!

The other way that I could tell Julie was a legit and honest breeder was that she asked me for a fifty-dollar deposit. That's all! Not fifty percent or eighty percent! Nothing like that. She asked for a fifty-dollar down payment and then the balance on delivery day, which is exactly how it is supposed to be. I, however, chose to e-transfer her the entire amount of the puppy. I know, it's really not recommended that you do that, but I had a really good feeling about Julie, so I just did it, and hoped that I wasn't going to regret it.

Soon came the day to "pick your puppy"! This happens around the six weeks old mark. Oh my gracious! I really never thought it would be so stressful! It was a Thursday, late afternoon. The puppies had coloured collars on and that's how they were identified.

Now, there is an order when it comes to who gets to pick first, then second, and so on. And I had no clue where I was on the list. I knew I wasn't at the very top of the list, but I didn't think I was at the very bottom either.

So, not really knowing how to do it, I looked at the puppies that Julie had put on her website, and I would pick the one that I liked, and then I would text Julie and ask if he was available. She would text me back and say, "No, sorry, he's already gone," or worse yet, "Someone before you still has to choose, but I've got you covered, don't worry." What does that mean? I thought to myself.

Thursday turned into Friday, and it was the same thing. I was still getting turned down, puppy after puppy. Julie was sending me the same text message: "Don't worry about it, Brenda."

Don't worry about what? I was so confused!

Lucky's Way

When Sunday morning came and I had still not picked a puppy, I had resigned myself to the thought that I had gotten scammed! I thought Julie had taken my money, scammed me, and that Bob was going to be really, really angry! I had a severe migraine setting in, and I thought to myself, I'm going to give it one more chance, so I got on Julie's website to see where the puppy selection was at, only to find my worst nightmare confirmed!

On the website, the only puppies left were small females. I was not happy and really not impressed! I texted Julie, "What the hell is going on? The only puppies left are females! You know I want a male! *I'm not impressed!*" Within a minute of me sending that text message, Julie called me, laughing! I have to admit, I thought "the nerve of some people"!

"Oh my God, Brenda, I'm so sorry! I should have called you earlier but I just couldn't risk it." I had no idea what she was talking about. Julie continued, "I had to wait until all of the males from this litter were picked before I could tell you that your puppy was one that I personally hand-picked from a completely different litter. I knew exactly which puppy would be perfect for what you plan on using him for because he's so laid-back and relaxed. He's a big boy with a boxy square head. He's a week younger than this other litter, but way bigger, and he'll still come home the same week as the others because they'll be nine weeks and he'll be eight weeks. I'm sending you pictures now." With that news, all was forgiven.

When it came time to pick up Harold, Julie delivered the puppies to a designated area approximately three hours away. Thankfully, Bob was able to drive with me to pick him up. There was a girl there with a full-grown Irish Wolfhound, who was waiting for her second puppy, and that was the first time Bob had ever seen one, so he was somewhat shocked by the size of the dog. That made me laugh. No turning back now, sweetie!

When Julie handed Harold to me, I thought I would just magically feel better. That I would fall in love with Harold on the spot, training would begin, and that would be it! Poof, depression gone, and I'd be myself again. It didn't work that way. I was still struggling with depression since Doug died, and although I was *seriously* happy to welcome a new puppy into my life, I wasn't sure if I was ready to begin loving him yet.

To be completely honest, I was scared of falling in love with Harold and having something happen to him. I really didn't think I could handle that kind of grief again. It was the second-most painful experience in my life. Next only to my father passing away.

I'm really not one hundred percent sure when I actually allowed myself to love Harold. I only know that he never gave up on me. When I had a particularly bad day, he never left my side. If I had a spontaneously difficult few minutes, brought on by a memory of Doug or my dad, Harold would come over, get up on my lap, and drape himself across me, all the while keeping his face squarely in my face, occasionally giving me a wee little kiss on my nose.

The bigger Harold got, the more his comforting began to help me. He's the perfect size for me to wrap my arms around his neck and chest and just hug him tight. Quite often this brings out even more sobs, but it doesn't faze Harold at all. He stands there and takes it all in, always willing and always happy to help.

I give Harold full credit for helping me through my depression and making me feel whole again. He is really, really good at his job. Harold helps get me through a lot of things in my life. I sincerely love all my dogs, but Harold is my special boy. He's far more sensitive to me and my emotions.

My family is what I consider "non-affectionate" toward each other. I'm not really sure why that is. Our son Dylan is the only one who likes to hug everyone when he leaves and I personally really love it. He would also always pick Harold up like a baby when he was a puppy. Dylan would carry him around like that as long as he could, until Harold got too big to pick up.

It seems to have backfired on poor Dylan now. When he walks in the door, Harold runs to him full tilt, then catapults himself onto Dylan, almost in an attempt to jump into his arms. It's really too funny. Harold has no idea he weighs 180 pounds and stands 7'5" when he's on his hind legs. In consolation, Dylan will sit on the couch, and Harold will sit on his lap and attempt to position himself in such a way that it resembles cradling a baby.

The moral of this story, folks, is to be very careful of what you are teaching your giant breed dogs as puppies, because they really don't forget and it might just end up becoming a ridiculous position you and your dog put yourselves in when your dog is full-grown.

Anyhow, back to the affectionate behaviour…I am very affectionate and loving with my dogs. I'm always hugging and kissing them, telling them how much I love them and how proud I am of them. (I do tell my kids that I love them and that I'm proud of them as well!)

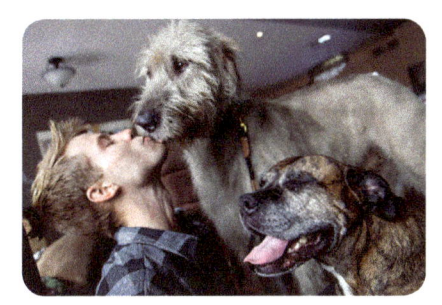

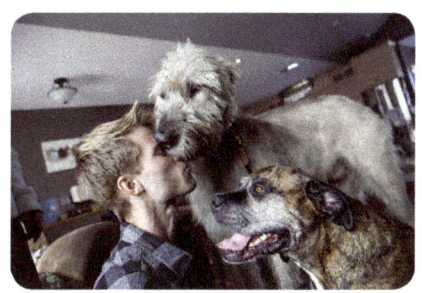

Dylan, Harold, and Hogan

DO NOT EVER BUY A PUPPY FROM A PET STORE!

Obviously, I can't stress this enough! **You will be getting a puppy from a puppy mill, with a whole host of problems.** Breeders don't sell their dogs to pet stores. They just don't. Not one reputable breeder I know would even consider selling a puppy to a pet store.

FINDING A PUPPY

Always buy a puppy from a reputable breeder who allows you to visit the puppy on-site so you can meet the mother (bitch) and, ideally, the father (stud or sire) as well. If the father is not on-site with the bitch, then the breeder should supply you with his address information so you can meet him if you choose to. In the case of the power breeds (for example, the Rottweiler, mastiff, German shepherd, pit bull, etc.), I would highly recommend that you take the time to visit the stud dog as well. You want to make sure that you know what temperament your puppy's parents are…both of them.

Oh, and since I brought up the pit bull breed, please do your homework before buying one of these powerful dogs. I am a huge believer in nurture over nature here, and I've spoken to many owners of pit bulls who agree that they are a very misjudged breed. Unfortunately, they can be very dangerous in the wrong hands and you must know how to properly train them to bring out the best in them. Also, there are counties in provinces across Canada where the pit bull breed is banned, and that is why, once again, *do your homework* so you don't end up with a dog who will end up being taken away from you in the long run.

There was a story on the news about a woman who had a pit bull as a family pet in her apartment. He had always been the most loving, sweet dog and had never shown any aggression whatsoever toward anyone, or any animal. Her dog apparently loved her longtime boyfriend, and therefore what happened seemed so out of character for the dog that the owner was completely shocked.

Her boyfriend had a grand mal seizure. He collapsed on the floor and was flailing about, and having never witnessed this before, the girlfriend was panic-stricken. Because of her anxiety, her usually sweet-natured pit bull was now feeding off the energy that she was giving off, and that sent him into protection mode.

It's instinctual with most dogs to protect their owners in times of danger and that's exactly what the pit bull thought was happening. He couldn't differentiate between a seizure and an attack. He just knew that something was terribly wrong and that his mistress needed help; he was going to give it the only way he knew how. Unfortunately, it ended in tragedy. Her loving, sweet-natured pit bull jumped in and mauled her boyfriend, ultimately killing him.

Had she remained calm, as some people do in emergency situations, I believe that her dog *might* have also remained calm, or, at the very least, calm enough that she could have removed him from the room in time to call 911. Most likely, in her dog's mind, he was only doing his job and saving her life.

That being said, I was not there, I did not witness this, and it is, of course, easy for me to sit back and say, "Remain calm in the face of an emergency," right? It was an awful situation, and my heart goes out to this lady, her family, and the family of her boyfriend.

Dogs, no matter what breed, will *always* fall back on their instincts. People need to understand that when deciding on a breed of dog. That is why, when you are choosing the breed you want, I can't stress enough that you do your homework. **My greatest fear is never what my dog could do to me, but what my dog could do to someone else... especially a child**. Please always keep that in mind.

STANDARD QUESTIONS THAT YOU SHOULD BE ASKING YOUR BREEDER:

Can I meet the parents? Or at least the bitch/mom? How old is the mom? (Does this make a difference? Not necessarily, but a healthy mom is an indication of how healthy the pups are, and if a breeder is still breeding a bitch into her senior years, that's a big red flag that the breeder is solely breeding for profit and not for quality, and personally, I would walk away from that kennel...actually, I'd run!)

Will the puppies be registered? If that matters to you, that is a question that needs to be asked because if the breeder is NOT a registered breeder with registered breeding stock, then you will not have a registered puppy...obviously. *FYI: Your dogs do not need to be registered with the Canadian Kennel Club or American Kennel Club to become registered service dogs or therapy dogs.

If you are purchasing a pup from a reputable breeder and paying good money for it, there's a good chance your breeder will bring up something about a non-breeding contract or something similar, which means you cannot start breeding your dog and selling the puppies, or in the case of the male dogs, use them for studs.

My opinion on this: LEAVE THE BREEDING TO THE PROFESSIONALS!

Honestly, I did the breeding puppies gig and it's not all that it's cracked up to be. It's hard work and unless your dogs are registered, there's no money in it! It's a 24/7 commitment. True blue breeders are a breed of their own, God bless them. It takes so much dedication to produce the best of the best breed standards, keep up with health checks for both bitches and studs, the whelping, weaning, the finding of good homes and sometimes having to re-home puppies who don't work out after the initial placement...and then there's the nonstop answering of questions from the clients who purchase or "adopt" a dog from you, which sometimes come in the middle of the night because they're panicking over whatever emergency situation just can't wait until morning...Oh my goodness, I could go on forever! That's why I say leave the breeding to the professionals! They deserve every penny they earn from the puppies and they know how to handle the neurotic people.

I *Do Not* ever recommend using your dog for stud! They can end up with an entire crackpot of issues, (again, that is a technical term), including but not limited to... non stop howling or barking after the first time, being bitten or attacked by the female, being dragged around by the female dog while still locked together - can you imagine how painful that must be to the male dog? - urinating uncontrollably (my sister's dog would pee on the corners of her bed after... yuck!), emotional scarring and more.

I've been asked if I would stud my big boy Harold and I said only if we did it by artificial insemination and sent the frozen semen. And that's done through a veterinarian...again, leave it to the professionals.

AN UNFORTUNATELY TRUE STORY...
The summer before I had Harold neutered, I was approached by a young man who asked me if I would consider using Harold as a stud to breed with his dog. Now, this gentleman was a kind of sketchy-looking young man to begin with...but who am I to judge a book by its cover? For all I know, he could be a CEO, right? Although if that were the case, in my humble opinion, I would suggest he pull his pants up over his skinny, five-and-a-half-foot-tall, underwear-exposed buttocks, and then, possibly, change out of that lovely, off-white bordering on dull grey, stained wife-beater shirt that read "Nice New Girlfriend - What Breed is She?" and into something less offensive.

Maybe I am a bit snobby? I've never really considered myself a snob, or even close to one, but good glory almighty, this guy rubbed me the wrong way right from the start, and it wasn't long before it got worse... much, much worse!

Lucky's Way

I asked him about the dog he wanted to breed with my 160-pound Irish Wolfhound (Harold was only a year old at this point). This is where it started to go sideways, I'm afraid.

"She's a nine-month-old Boston Terrier," he said, straight-faced.

Now, it seriously took me a minute to get my brain wrapped around what this idiot had just said to me!

"I'm sorry, did you just say a Boston I mean, maybe it's just me? Terrier?" I asked, hoping that I had somehow blacked out or seriously misheard him!

"Oh yeah, man! I've been, like, looking for a, like, big dog to, like, breed her with, so she can have, like, some super cool puppies, dude. Don't you, like, think that would be, like, so f'ing awesome?"

At this point, my left eye started to twitch. Never a good sign!

"Yeah, no, dude! I do not *like* think that would be *like* f'ing awesome! Do you not have *like* a brain in your f'ing head, dude? Think about this for a minute! If, just if, you actually find someone stupid enough to breed a giant dog with your female, not only would it be like you getting raped by a 300-pound football player, but, and here's a BIG BUT so please pay close attention, God forbid she got pregnant, those puppies, just growing inside her, would be so big she'd probably rip apart! And if! IF! she somehow didn't die between the breeding and the pregnancy, she'd definitely have to have a scheduled c-section, which would cost you a small fortune! Good Lord, son! Have you asked your vet about any of this? Surely your vet would have told you this is not a good idea! Did they give you a quote on a c-section? Actually, I don't even care if you have the money; it's just way too cruel to put your dog through that! Seriously, what did your vet say when you told them what you were planning?"

The look on his face was priceless. "Hey? Dude? I asked you a question!" I was looking at his face and he'd actually gone pale.

"Umm, yeah, sorry, lady, like, slow down, I'm still kinda, like, stuck on the whole raping thing so I, like, didn't really hear anything you said after that."

Oh Lord! I actually had to repeat it to him all over again! But thankfully, THANKFULLY, I think I finally got through to him.

The moral of the story...Please, PLEASE, leave the breeding to the professionals!

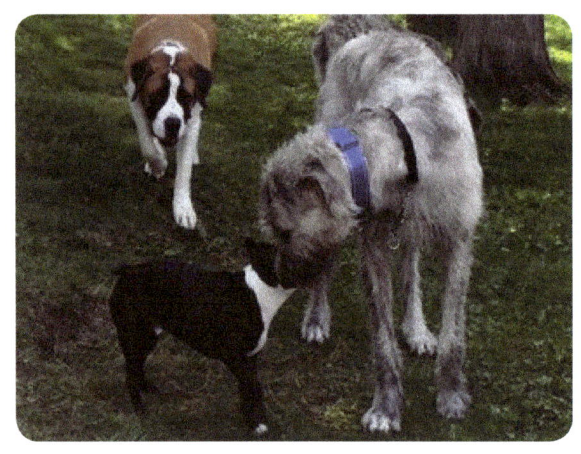

This is not the Boston Terrier depicted in the story (this one happens to be a male), I just wanted to give you a visual. Can you even imagine?!

Anyway, onward...

AT WHAT AGE WILL I GET MY PUPPY?

You should get the puppy at eight to ten weeks old, depending on the breed of dog.

WILL MY PUPPY HAVE ANY SHOTS WHEN I GET THEM?

Some breeders now offer a choice when it comes to first shots. Personally, I'm still old-school and believe in getting my dogs vaccinated and if the breeder is willing to pay for the first set, that's a bonus.

Depending on the breed of dog, you may need to talk to your breeder about docking tails or cropping ears. These are breed-specific practices; although to some people they may seem very cruel, it's what the breed standard calls for. If this is something you are completely uncomfortable with, talk to your breeder and see if they'll leave your puppy's tail and/or ears intact. If they won't and that's a deal-breaker, well, then I guess the only option would be to look for a different breeder or possibly even choose a different breed of dog altogether.

Dew claws may fall into this category as well, which is another discussion to have with both breeder and veterinarian if it is a concern.

DOES MY PUPPY COME WITH A HEALTH GUARANTEE?

If you're getting your pup from a kennel, as opposed to a backyard breeder, they should offer some form of health guarantee, so feel free to bring it up if it's not something that is brought up by them.

IS MY PUPPY MICROCHIPPED?

Backyard breeders are not going to microchip your puppy for you, whereas a registered breeder is almost guaranteed to sell you a puppy that has both, the health guarantee and the microchip. In either case, your vet can do one or both for you if that's your wish.

HOW MUCH SHOULD YOU PAY FOR A PUPPY?

Here, again, is where you really have to do your homework! There's absolutely nothing wrong with some, *some*, backyard breeders. You have to check them out and be sure to follow through on meeting the parents and such.

My advice would be, spending $1,200 on a backyard, unregistered, un-microchipped, no-health-guarantee dog is probably what I would consider to be my maximum budget. I've spent way less on one. Hemi, for example, was $600 and both parents were on site (yes, I bought my son his dog).

I'll give you a few examples, so you'll have some numbers to work with. Lloyd was $800; Truman (another big Saint Bernard, now deceased) was $600; Clark, my new Saint Bernard, cost me $1,000. Earl, a harlequin Great Dane, was $1200 from a registered breeder; however, he was not registered with the CKC. He ended up going blind (he had sky-blue eyes, which was not breed-specific, and I did not know that at the time), and because of that, he got really mean and nasty and he had to be put down by the age of three. For Irish Wolfhounds, depending on the breeder, you're going to pay anywhere from $1,800–$5,000 or more. The best dog we've had on our farm was Bud; he was a Rottweiler/Lab cross and I paid $75 for him. Best money I ever spent!

Never, ever send the breeder the full purchase amount via internet payment! Any reputable breeder only asks for a percentage to secure your puppy and full payment is made when you pick your pup up. That's pretty standard procedure.

GIANT DOG BREED DEFINITION

Giant dog breeds are defined by both size and weight. A giant breed is over one hundred pounds and stands at a shoulder height of 26" and above.

Here is a list of the top ten giant breed dogs:

- Irish Wolfhound
- Saint Bernard
- Great Dane
- Mastiff
- Leonberger
- Bullmastiff
- Newfoundland
- Dogue de Bordeaux
- Great Pyrenees
- Neapolitan Mastiff

THINGS YOU SHOULD KNOW BEFORE BUYING A GIANT BREED DOG

Whenever I'm out with any of them, especially Harold and Leonard, I get asked the same question over and over again: "How much did you pay for them?"

Firstly, I think it's rude to ask someone that, call me crazy (many have); it rates right up there with "How much money do you make?" or "How much do you weigh?" (kind of personal questions), but I do answer, with a smile, and really, really *wish* I could say something like, "Seriously? Are you really that rude? If you're seriously interested in the breed then do your homework and find a breeder and ask them how much a puppy costs!" But instead I hold my smile and give, between clenched teeth, the same reply: "The initial cost of the puppy is the cheapest part of owning a giant breed dog."

In this day and age of technology, when you can google darn near everything, there's really no need to ask such a personal question. My own husband doesn't even know exactly how much I've paid for some of my dogs. So please, if you are one of *those* people, *STOP* doing that! Now, let's get back to it.

When you own a giant breed, everything is giant: the food bills, the vet bills, the grooming fees, etc. Not only do giant breed dogs come with giant breed costs like giant food costs, giant vet bills, giant grooming fees (if needed), they also need giant amounts of room to grow and a giant-size bed as well as giant-sized toys, giant-sized dishes and a giant amount of exercise. It's always a good idea to consult a vet and ask, before you buy a giant breed dog, how much it will cost to get them neutered or spayed. Again, responsible dog ownership is key here.

DOGS AND EXERCISE

All dogs need exercise, from the minis to the giant breeds! They all need to go for walks every day—twice a day would benefit them the most. It's a misnomer that the bigger the breed, the less exercise it needs. It is true that some dogs are definitely more energetic than others, but regardless, ALL DOGS NEED EXERCISE!

Ask your breeder, the adoption agency, or your vet if you are unsure of exactly how much exercise your particular dog needs. It's better to know ahead of time if you're looking at a high-energy breed like the Australian shepherd or at something more low-key, like a Neapolitan mastiff.

Just today my husband told me to stop buying toys for our dogs. I asked him why and he told me that he's been noticing that there are actually pieces of rope, stuffing material, etc. in the dog poop that's lovingly left either on our driveway or the lawn.

I'm fairly certain it's Leonard, my younger Wolfhound, eating these things right now and I can't imagine why. Other than that, he's cute as a button and smart like dump truck (that's one of our favourite sayings when we refer to our dogs doing "not so brilliant" things).

One more thing while on the subject of giant breeds and what to expect… big disasters! Quite possibly HUGE destruction! I've heard of some dogs chewing couches, entire bathrooms or laundry rooms if they are locked in for long periods of time, walls (thank you, Clark Griswald), dining room tables, and any kind of wooden furniture seems to be fair game for giant breeds.

Leonard seems to love ripping apart full boxes of Kleenexes! Why? I just don't get it. It's the cardboard that he rips up, so the tissues are spewed everywhere! Oh, and don't get me started on the eating of underwear! Seriously! What is with that? A lack of cotton in their systems? Crazy freaking dogs!

For Harold it's blankets; he has to pull every blanket off every couch, chair, stool, whatever, wherever there may be one, and pull it onto the floor. Sometimes this results in a tug of war between some of the dogs, so bye bye blanket, otherwise it's just dog hair city and that lovely eau de dog scent they leave behind.

My point here is to be aware of what you are possibly getting yourself into with not just any dog, but from a tiny one to a giant one.

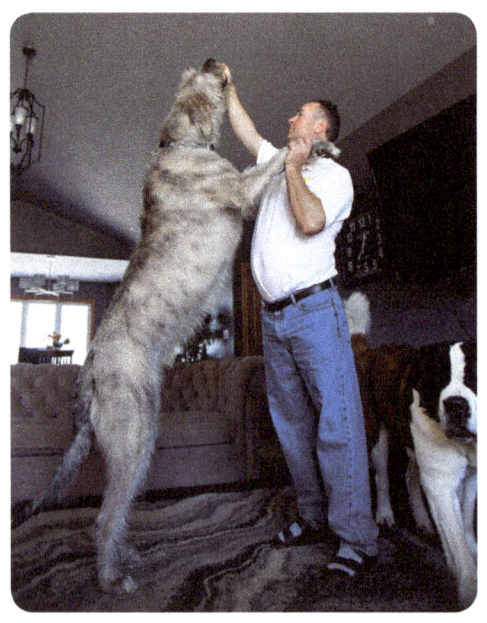

Harold is seven feet five inches tall and Bob is six feet four inches tall

ALL VETERINARIANS ARE NOT CREATED EQUAL
Finding the Right One For You and Your Dog

Before you even get your puppy or new dog, find a vet. It's very important to have a good relationship with your vet. You have to be able to trust them. How do you find the right vet for you? Ask around! Ask your friends who have dogs, ask your neighbours, if they have dogs, heck, ask the people who walk past your house with their dogs!

If you don't already have a veterinarian that you use and trust, price around and don't let them talk you into unnecessary stuff. If you're unsure of what they're trying to sell you, tell them you're going to think about it, and again, ask around. Ask your friends with dogs if they've had this or that done and if it is something worth looking into for your dog.

After you find your new vet, ask some important questions about your new dog's potential health costs. How much will first immunizations cost? How much does flea, tick, and worm protection cost annually? How much will it cost to spay or neuter your dog? Dog food recommendations, etc?

One more thing to remember: a *good* vet will only *recommend* things to you that you actually need; a *great* vet will not only look out for your pet, but also your wallet, and not bulls**t you into poverty.

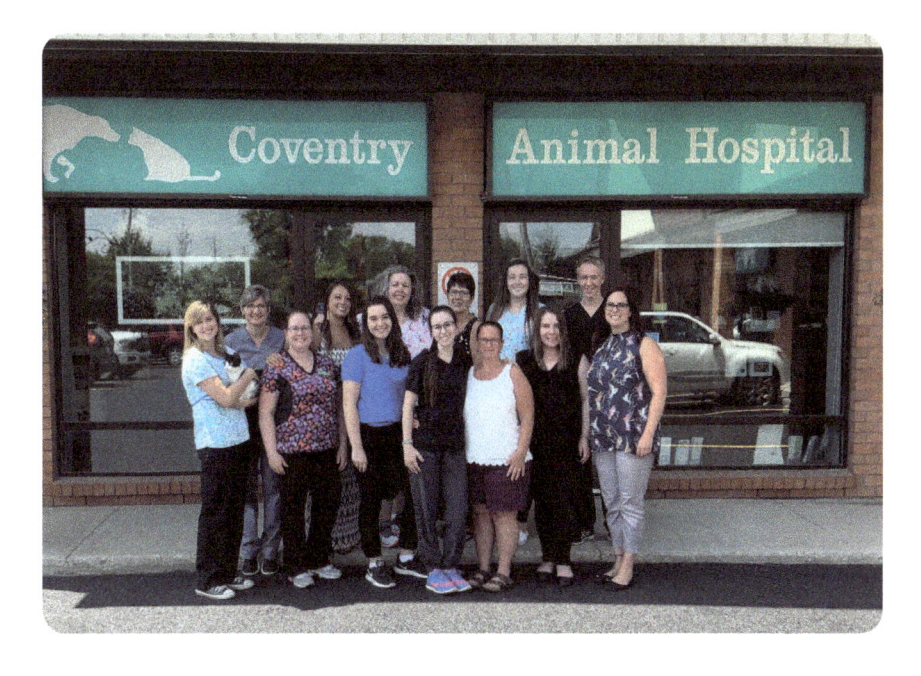

Brenda Boemer-Groenestege

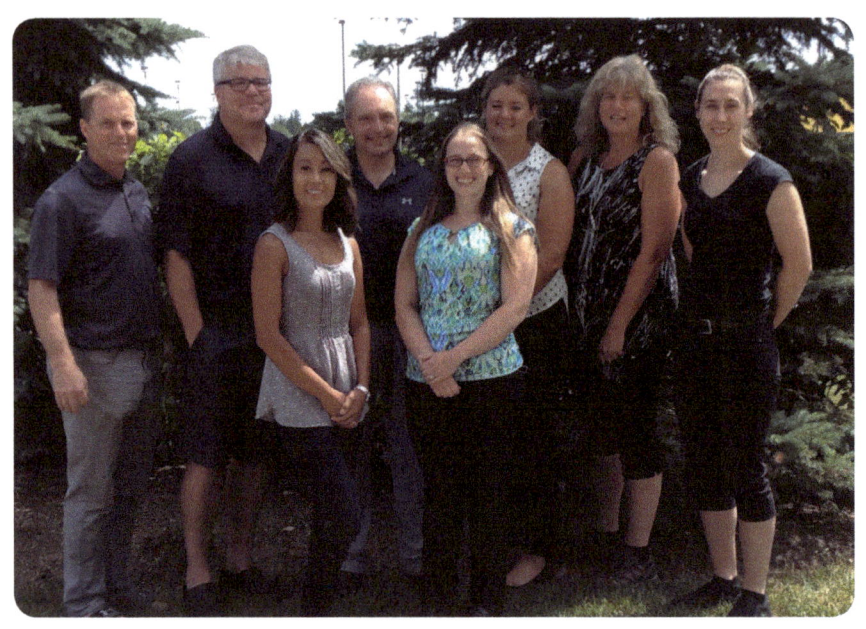

The best team of Veterinarians, Veterinary Technicians, office staff, full & part-time staff, and even their office mascot (an adorable three-legged cat named Charm) make every visit enjoyable for you and your pet.

Case in point:

In August 2018, Hemi, my grand-dog, needed a lump removed from her ear. They quoted me one price, listing everything that they would be doing that day, which included blood work to check for thyroid abnormalities because she had gained four pounds in two months.

When the surgery was finished and I came to pick her up, Dr. Angela filled me in on how smoothly the surgery went and (here's where the *great* vet title comes in) she proceeded to tell me that because it went so well and unexpectedly quickly (something she absolutely did not have to tell me because I would never have been the wiser), it brought the cost down to $600.00, close to half the quoted price!

Amazing, right? Plus, initially they thought she would probably need to be on antibiotics after the surgery, and again, because of how clean and noninvasive the surgery was, no antibiotics! So, no extra money handed out.

Oh, and did I mention they trimmed her nails for FREE as well?! I've said it before and I'll say it again…I have the best vet clinic team in the whole wide world! I love, Love, LOVE them!

Their commitment, professionalism, honesty, integrity, customer loyalty and service, and, of course, their genuine love of pets giant or extra small, makes them a GREAT veterinary clinic in my books. Oh, and they will do house calls in emergency situations! AMAZING, RIGHT?!

Thank you, Dr. Angela Gerretsen, D.V.M., and Dr. Glenn Armstrong, D.V.M., and staff at Coventry in Stratford and Mitchell Veterinary. Love you guys!

CHAPTER 6

And So the Training Begins

BRINGING YOUR PUPPY HOME

Whether you're planning on using your puppy for therapy or not, every puppy needs to start basic training and be housebroken as soon as possible. The minute that puppy comes home, the training starts.

You need to decide who is going to be the alpha in the family. Is it going to be you? Your partner or spouse? Or even possibly one of your children, if they are responsible and commanding enough? It absolutely, positively, cannot be your dog or you're screwed right off the bat!

Sorry, this is not one of those training manuals where we do not use the word "no." There is actually a dog training class out there somewhere in Ontario where they refuse to use "NO" in their puppy training class. They believe it's inhumane and that you should compromise with your dog. I'm not even sure how that's possible, to be honest.

The mother of a girl who was enrolled in such a class was telling me all about how terribly her daughter's King shepherd (110 pounds and 28" tall) was trained. She explained that every time she comes home with him, he literally lunges…not jumps but runs, dragging his owner behind him, and lunges up onto her, knocking her down, and that several times she has had some pretty bad injuries.

He has also given her daughter, his owner, some fairly nasty injuries because of this ridiculous type of training! Her mother begged me for help, which I, of course, offered wholeheartedly. Since then, her daughter has seen the beauty in saying "NO"!

Reprimanding your dog, when needed, is a sign of being an alpha dog. With the King shepherd, obviously he was still the alpha and his owner needed to take that role back as soon as possible!

HOUSE TRAINING MADE EASY

Every dog has what I like to call a "TELL" when they have to go to the bathroom. It's normally more visible when they have to go poop, but it's there; you just have to *pay attention.* Some will sniff around intensely, maybe in a circle, or whimper a bit, and then you'll notice their butt starting to squat, or some may lift their tail in the air, or some even start to back up...whatever it is, try to figure it out and it will make housebreaking so much easier.

After every nap, put your puppy outside on the grass, because they need to pee, and use your words: "Go pee pee, puppy." Getting your dog used to hearing you give them that command will come in very handy in the future if you're traveling with them or if you decide to train them as a therapy dog and need them to use the break time to go outside on the grass and do their business in a limited amount of time.

Every time your puppy successfully accomplishes his business outside you must praise him with lots and lots of verbal and physical love and encouragement.

This sometimes takes a bit of time too, folks, so patience is key here. Don't expect your puppy to run outside and do their bathroom business immediately every time. Just like for humans, sometimes it may take a few minutes, especially if the weather is poor outside. I know for a fact that my own dogs hate it when it's freezing-cold rain. They stick their head out the door and then retreat back and look at me as if they are saying, "Oh, heck no, Mom, I'm not going out in that! Are you kidding?" Then they wait until they absolutely cannot hold it any longer, and then they run outside and do what needs to be done as fast as possible.

Unfortunately, puppies don't quite have the same willpower as more mature dogs, and therefore will end up doing their bathroom business on your floor if you don't wait outside with them until they have managed to get everything done out there. I find it's really handy to have one of those nice big golf umbrellas around; it keeps the weather off you and your puppy.

Lucky's Way

Whether it's the spring, summer, fall, or winter, potty training is the same. The only difference is that your puppy, depending on breed, probably won't want to stand outside in the freezing cold any longer than you do. Nonetheless, patience is still the key here. Bundle up, folks, you and your puppy! If it's cold for you, it's cold for them, especially if they are a short-haired breed. And please remember their little feet! You wear big heavy boots to keep your feet warm in the winter months, but some of the tiny teacup breeds can freeze very quickly, so be mindful of that.

Now, if your puppy has accidents in the house, normally it's because you weren't paying attention, or were just being plain old lazy and didn't bother getting up in time to put the puppy out. In any case, don't give the dog too much grief for it; maybe say something like, "Oh no, puppy goes poop outside" and leave it at that. It was an accident, after all. I'm sure you have heard that old saying, "Don't sweat the small stuff"? Well, that is very important for you to remember when your puppy is at that very destructive, rotten, accident-prone stage in its life. It is short-lived, even though it can seem like a lifetime.

I'm a huge believer in training without treats, because you're not always going to have treats with you when you want your dog to do something (like come to you if he ran off at the park) but you'll always have lots of love, hugs, and kisses to give him, right? And if, by chance, you do have treats with you on occasion, well, that's just a bonus for your dog. However, some dogs do much better when enticed with treats, especially when they are puppies and therefore I tend to use treats when I am beginning their training. Teaching your dog to respond to commands strictly when given a treat isn't the best habit to form, so slowly hold off on always rewarding with treats and reward with lots of love and praise as an alternative.

Don't get me wrong, my boys sure know the word "treat" because, come on, they are completely spoiled rotten after all. They will do almost anything for one, but I try to only use treats if they really deserve them… like, did they actually do what I asked of them immediately? For example, did they drop the barn cat out of their mouth and get their butts in the house as soon as I told them to? That kind of thing.

CRATE TRAINING: DO I OR DON'T I?

Yes is the short answer; crate training can save your house and your marriage. Okay, I'll come clean. I, for one, do not crate my puppy at night because I like to cuddle him in my bed! Oh, I can hear the gasps.

I know, bad Brenda! Bad, bad Brenda! It is a completely selfish thing to do on my part, but I do it because I can. Look, folks, this is something that I feel is a personal preference and therefore I am completely unapologetic about it!

I actually just bought myself a king-sized bed. Thankfully, Clark is not a huge fan of sleeping in the bed with me, because it's too hot or maybe too crowded since Harold, Leonard, and Lloyd sleep with me as well.

Where's my husband, Bob, you may be asking? Coincidentally, I'm going through—cue the voice of God—*the change of life*! And therefore I'm sleeping in the spare bedroom with the fan on high and the window open in the cooler months or closed during air conditioning months, yet I'm still managing to sweat through my pjs a couple times a night. So hubby gets the master bedroom with a king-sized bed to himself, and I now also have a king-sized bed, hot flashes, and four dogs…whatever, it works for us. TMI, I know, sorry about that.

Okay, back to crate training. Crates for giant-breed dogs can be very challenging to find and extraordinarily expensive. Besides, most will grow out of their crate by the time they're five or six months old or even sooner.

Crate training for any other size dog, from a teacup size to a large breed, is highly recommended. Not only does the crate help prevent accidents and damage while you are away at work, but some dogs will become very attached to their crate and enjoy having their own space. Allowing them to have their own place where no one is allowed to bother or pester them is very important, especially if there are young children in the home or visiting often.

This brings up a very important point: when you have company over and you know that your puppy or dog might feel overwhelmed, putting them in their safe place (i.e., their crate) will allow them to feel calm in an otherwise stressful situation. However, make sure your company, especially if there are little ones, know that your puppy or dog is off-limits for the duration of the party. Setting firm boundaries is always very important

Lucky's Way

for the well-being of not only your dog, but your guests as well. If they end up sticking their hands into the dog's safety zone, it could end poorly for both dog and guest, and no one wants that.

A dog's crate is their safe haven. If they feel cornered, especially if it's during a party or a loud get-together, where they can't necessarily see you for reassurance, and a stranger, whether a child or adult, intrudes on their safe space by sticking their hand into that space, well, it's fight or flight for some dogs.

Now, what happens next? Well, if the dog has a chance to get out of the crate without getting "caught" by this stranger, that's most likely what your dog will try to do, thank goodness. In some instances, however, when that's not possible, the dog will give proper warning by cowering, then giving low, guttural growls in hopes that the stranger backs off. When that doesn't work, well, that adult or child will get bit. In the case of the adult, we say, "Well, you were told not to bug the dog," but in the case of the child, it gets a lot more challenging. As the owner of the dog, you want to yell at the parents, "WHERE THE HELL WERE YOU? And why were you not watching your kids?" But this is where being a responsible dog owner comes into play.

Let's rewind the situation. You are having a party. You put your puppy or dog in its crate and put that crate behind a **LOCKED** door, so this never happens. This could be your bedroom, your garage, or, heck, even ask your parents or a friend to babysit.

Thinking of your dog as a child is not crazy. What would you do to keep your child safe? The better question is, what wouldn't you do, right?

The other benefit of using a crate is, obviously, the potty training. It's not rocket science: after your puppy eats, put him outside because he needs to poop. After your puppy wakes up from a nap, put your puppy outside for a pee. After your puppy has a big drink, put your puppy outside for a pee. If your puppy has been in the crate for a while, put your puppy outside for a pee or poop. First thing in the morning…well, that's just obvious, I hope, but you get the drift, right? And when your puppy does go pee or poo outside, lots of praise from you.

NIGHTTIME SOOTHING

Sometimes your puppy just doesn't want to be alone. Think about it from your puppy's perspective for a minute or two before you lose your mind and your temper, okay? From the time your puppy is born, they are surrounded by their mom and multiple siblings, as well as, usually, adoring human beings. And now they are singled out, on their own, alone, in a crate at night. Of course they're crying. Wouldn't you be?

One idea to help make the transition a little easier for your puppy and to help him get settled and soothed at night is the old put-an-alarm-clock-under-his-bed trick. Just make sure it's one that makes a pretty loud ticking sound; it mimics the sound of his mother's heartbeat. Also, if you put a mirror beside his crate, he can see his "twin" beside him. I've heard that has worked for a lot of puppy owners.

I'm a firm believer in treating your puppy like you would a new baby for the first little while. If they are really beside themselves at night, my number-one suggestion is to bring the crate into your bedroom.

When your puppy starts to whine, talk soothingly to him/her. If the crate is close enough, reach over and rub his head and tell him, "It's okay, hush, it's nighttime." Just like with children, this will not last forever. If it helps you and your pup sleep through the night, I say, Amen, and do it. Do whatever works to get you sleeping through the night.

As far as giving the puppy food and water after a certain time of night, I would definitely put up his water dish around seven to eight o'clock, depending on your schedule; this way he really shouldn't need to pee until morning.

On a personal note, I have found that the heavier breeds, like my Saint Bernards, really find it difficult to self-regulate their body heat, and therefore I'm up and down with Clark Griswald multiple times during the night just so he can go outside and cool off. Truman was the exact same way. They need to go outside and lie down in the snow for around twenty minutes and then they want back inside. Doesn't this irritate you, you ask? Hell yes! But I love my dogs and therefore I do what needs to be done to keep them happy and healthy.

TRAINING YOUR DOG TO DRINK FROM A WATER BOTTLE
No gimmicks needed

This may sound silly, but I assure you that it is one skill that will come in very handy. Teaching your puppy to drink from a water bottle at a young age can be a lifesaver!

Your puppy will very quickly pick up on this trick. Begin by gently pouring water from the bottle into your hand, allowing your puppy to drink it, but making sure your pup is feeling the end of the water bottle. Practicing this while your pup is young will ensure a life long ability to stay hydrated for both you and your dog as long as you remember to bring along the water bottles. It comes in very handy when we are out and about and I don't have a bowl for water. I can buy a bottle (or six) of water for my guys and they get hydrated without pulling out anything like a popup water bowl or any other gimmick. Given a choice, my dogs will drink from a tap or water bottle instead of a bowl of water every time.

Tip: fill a water bottle two thirds full with water; put that in the freezer and allow it to freeze fully, then give that to your puppy or dog on a hot summer day! This works well for puppies who are teething (and babies too!!).

LET'S TALK FOOD AND DOG TREATS

The amount of different kinds of dog food on the market today is overwhelming, so I could never choose one dog food alone to recommend. Not when there are so many wonderful brands out there.

First, ask your breeder what they would recommend for your new puppy. If, by chance, that food isn't available to you or isn't in your budget, go into your local pet store and ask them for their recommendation. Let them know both your breed of dog and your budget and I guarantee you that they will be more than willing to find a dog food brand for you.

WHAT TO LOOK FOR IN YOUR DOG'S FOOD

Ingredients such as blueberries, blackberries, pomegranate, or raspberries indicate that the dog food is likely rich with antioxidants. These help boost the immune system and accelerate the healing process. Omega-3 and omega-6 fatty acids from flaxseed and salmon oil help produce a shiny coat, while mixed tocopherols and rosemary extract act as natural preservatives. Salmon oil and turmeric together provide anti-inflammatory properties that help your dog's mobility.

The first ingredient should always be protein of some sort, whether chicken, pork, beef, or salmon. Eggs and meat meals have high bioavailability for dogs. These sources of protein have amino acids and are easy for dogs to digest.

This may sound confusing, but healthy alternatives that you want to look for in your dog's food are "whole grains" or "grain free." Choose nutritious whole grains such as quinoa, oats, or brown rice, OR ditch the grains and choose a natural grain-free dog food.

Avoid artificial colours in dog food and dog treats. They may look visually appealing, but they have been linked to hyperactivity in dogs, as well as several biochemical processes within the body. They are completely unnecessary!

Another ingredient to look for is salt. Salt is necessary for humans and dogs alike, but too much salt is harmful to both of you. Always keep an eye on the salt in your pet's food and treats.

Most pet stores will send home sample bags of dog food for your pup to try to see which one they like. This way you don't have to worry about spending money on a bag of dog food for your dog and having him not like it.

Locally, we have a couple of amazing pet stores: Global Pet Foods and PetValu. Both have equally knowledgeable staff and amazing service. I have them both on speed dial. It's comforting to know that when I call Cole at Global to order my dog food for the month, it's going to be ready for pick-up as soon as I get there. Plus, he does all the heavy lifting for me. I love that guy!

If you are looking into getting a giant breed puppy, then you will need to feed him/her "large breed puppy food,"

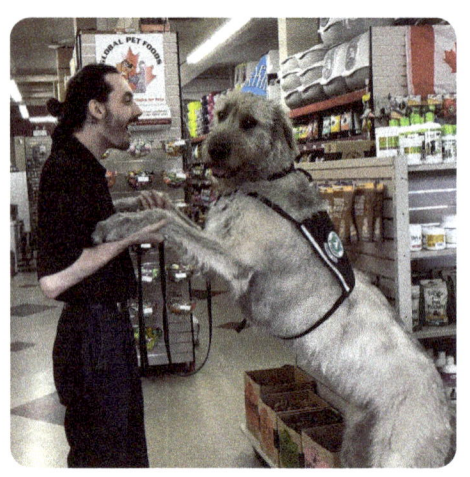

Cole dancing with Harold

Lucky's Way

which has everything that your giant breed pup needs for healthy growth. My vets still recommend that I keep my boys on a combination of half adult and half puppy large breed food. This is personal preference. What works for me and my dogs may not work for other dogs. Check with your vet and or ask your breeder or the adoption facility where you received your dog.

If you have a senior dog, or an overweight dog, then you want to look for that specific type of dog food for your dog. Small dogs need kibble made for them as well. Quite often with the smaller breeds, your vet may recommend that you mix wet dog food with the dry kibble so your little dog finds it easier to eat. As well, giving your little guy multiple smaller meals in a day, rather than one big meal once a day, is much easier on their digestion.

Feeding multiple smaller meals in a day can be used for all sizes and breeds of dogs if you find your dog is hungry all the time, or if, right after you feed them, they throw up their big meal. Some dogs tend to eat really, really quickly, and therefore they aren't actually chewing or digesting their food before it hits their stomach, which means that they end up throwing it up again soon after eating it. If this sounds familiar, I would recommend that you feed your dog multiple smaller meals in a day and buy him a "Gobble Stopper" or "slow feed" dog food bowl (you can find these online from $7.99 to $44.99 depending on the size of the bowl). These bowls are made to prevent your dog from eating super-fast and thus give the food time to actually digest. They also give your dog some mental stimulation, which is always good.

When you bring your pup home, your breeder will most likely send along some of the puppy food that they were eating to incorporate into the new brand so it doesn't upset their tummy. When picking puppy food, you want to look for one that has omega-3 fatty acids listed on the ingredients; this ingredient helps support normal cognitive development in your puppy.

It's a good idea to mix a bit of warm water with your puppy's food to soften it up for the first week or two, since your little one still has very small teeth and even puppy kibble can be a challenge to break apart.

If your puppy has loose stools when he first comes home, *you need to take a stool sample in to your vet* to get it checked for worms. This is very, very common in puppies. A natural remedy for loose stools is pumpkin purée (not pumpkin pie filling). Just mix a couple tablespoons in with their food and that should help tighten things up.

However, if they have worms, only worm medication can help get rid of them. The majority of puppies do have worms. It doesn't matter if you got your puppy from the most exclusive breeder in the world, there's still a ninety-nine percent chance that it will have worms! They get them from the mother through her milk. So, please, please, if your puppy has the runs, take a sample to your vet's office ASAP and get it checked out!

ALLERGIES AND DOG FOOD

If you have determined that your dog has a food allergy, I would recommend feeding him Kangaroo kibble. Dogs I know who have specific skin problems who switched to Kangaroo kibble have done amazingly well. It may be a little hard to find, so ask your vet.

RAW FOOD DIET

What is a raw food diet and what are the pros and cons of it? The raw food diet started with greyhounds and sled dogs. It was suggested that dogs would flourish when fed a raw food diet, also known as the BARF diet, which stands for *Bones and Raw Food* or *Biologically Appropriate Raw Food*.

Raw dog food consists of uncooked meat, usually organ and muscle meat, whole or crushed bones, vegetables, raw eggs, fruits, and some dairy products.

Pros of the Raw Food Diet:

- Shinier coat
- Healthier skin
- Cleaner teeth
- More energy
- smaller stools

Cons of the Raw Food Diet:

- Very expensive

- Bacteria in the raw meat poses a threat to human health if meat is not handled properly.

- Giving whole bones to dogs poses a risk of internal punctures, broken teeth, and choking.

For more information about the raw food diet, check out Canine Journal online at caninejournal.com. I found it to be a great source of not only information about the raw food diet, but recipes and more.

TREATS: SOMETIMES YOU JUST HAVE TO SPOIL THEM

It was brought to my attention recently that a dog nearly died because of treats that came from a dollar store. This, unfortunately, doesn't surprise me. Most dogs love treats; however, the wrong treats can be deadly for them. Going into a trusted pet food store or your vet clinic and asking their opinion on which treats they recommend is always the best idea.

Some dog treats can also be quite expensive, which is another reason I'm glad that I was taught to train with praise and not treats. Buying in bulk and storing treats safely will save you money in the long run. Another trick I like is buying the bigger treats and cutting them into smaller portions. It seems that we are always paying extra for the tiny treats, when the same ones in a bigger size can cost less and be cut down into bite-size pieces for training or snacking purposes.

If using treats for training, use the dried liver treats, they are versatile and can be snapped into any size for any dog. The other treats you will always find in my pantry are called "Greenies." They are in the shape of a toothbrush. They can be bought economically in a supersized pack and they are quite large, so they can be cut down quite a bit if that's what works for you and your budget.

LET'S TALK HOT SPOTS

This topic was new to me, believe it or not. Exactly what is a hot spot? A hot spot is an infected area of inflamed skin that is very uncomfortable for your dog. Hot spots are caused by a condition called acute moist dermatitis. They become itchy, irritable, painful skin lesions that become worse by constant licking, biting, chewing and scratching at the infected area. The inflammation causes these spots to become warm, or "hot" which is how they got their name.

Shortly after a freak two-day rainstorm, Clark presented with what initially looked like a bloody back, as if he'd gotten into a brawl with one of my other dogs. But when I tried to touch him, he cried out in pain, even when I tried to move his fur. I knew something was very, very wrong.

I rushed Clark to the vet clinic, where he was sedated, and, to my absolute horror, the top half of his back was revealed to be an explosion of one gigantic bloody, infected hot spot. I was shocked! How on earth could this happen?

How did I miss this? Well, the answer is, Clark and Harold roughhouse when they play, and the vet found a little puncture mark on Clark's back, right behind his collar. She explained that that one little puncture wound and forty-eight hours of rain was the perfect combination to make the infection grow and fester.

Clark has very thick, dense, curly hair. When he came in from the rain, I didn't think to dry him off, so the dampness kept the infection on his back in the perfect state to spread, and it finally exploded into a painful mess of blood and pus. Talk about mom guilt! I still feel awful about it!

There are other reasons for dogs to get hot spots, including food allergies, anxiety, heat, fabric softener allergies, and more.

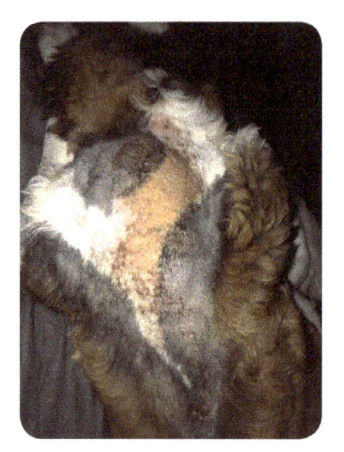

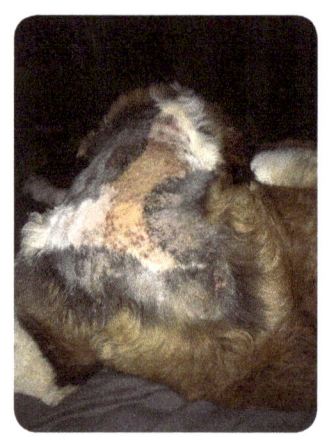

Clark Griswald's crazy big hot spot!

TRAINING: WHAT EVERY DOG AND OWNER SHOULD KNOW
Engaging Mental Stimulation

One question that I get asked quite frequently is, "How do I train my puppy or dog to stay out of the garbage, or stop destroying things in my home?"

Your puppy or dog is trying to tell you that he's bored! Yes, that is a thing! Dogs get bored all the time and need to be stimulated and engaged, not only physically but mentally as well.

Taking your dog for a long walk is great exercise and will help tire them out, but giving them something that is mentally challenging, especially while you have gone to work or gone out for a while, ticks both boxes. It exercises the mind and body.

A "treat ball" is made of hard rubber with holes in it where the treats come out as your dog moves it around with its paw or nose. This type of treat toy comes in all shapes and sizes, just like dogs.

I am quite sure that the crafty people out there could probably make something like this. Pinterest is a great source of ideas here. I've seen treat toys made using empty cardboard milk or juice containers. The only issue can be that, if left alone with the empty container, your puppy or dog may decide to rip it apart and even eat it, so be very careful. If you use homemade treat containers like this, make sure you can be home with your dog to supervise.

One of my favourite homemade treat containers is an almost empty peanut butter tub. Three out of four of my dogs love peanut butter, so when the jar is pretty much empty, I use a butter knife or spoon to smear peanut butter over the rest of the sides, then I break up some liver treats and push them into the sticky sides, and there you have it, a cheap and cheerful distraction. Make sure you peel off the paper label from the peanut butter container and any glue on the sides. And leave the lid off, unless your dog is really, really smart.

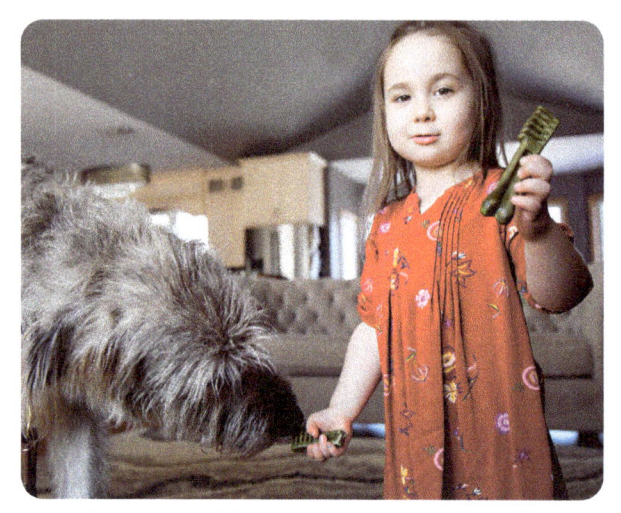

My great-niece Ayla using Greenies treats with Harold.

BASIC TRAINING

Training your puppy can start as soon as you decide you want to start putting the work into him or her. In my case, with my therapy dogs, it starts as soon as I get them home, at around eight weeks old. All dogs should learn the basics but there's one rule that I am adamant about and that is food or toy aggression—that's a huge no no in my books.

When your puppy comes home, the first time you put food down, get your hands in there with their food and see what that pup is like. If it growls or reacts aggressively, you need to act on it immediately!

AN AGGRESSIVELY TRUE STORY:

When I brought Harold home at eight weeks old, the very last thing I was expecting was that I would be getting a little bugger biter that decided to give me a run for my money on the second day he was home.

It started when my niece Mallory was over and I was showing off my new puppy. I gave Harold a toy and he snarled and snapped at my hand! Well, holy mother of pearl, I was not expecting that. Here I thought I had this super chill Irish Wolfhound, but he turned into a freaking Satan's child if you tried to take away a toy or, heaven forbid, a bone!

Well, that was not going to fly with this old bird! It was the fighting Irish against the stubborn German and not just for days but for weeks! I'm not going to lie; there was a point when I wondered if I'd ever get that aggression out of him. He was quite literally like Dr. Jekyll and Mr. Hyde, so sweet and loving one minute, but then wham, try to take away a toy or something and he's trying to take off your arm! I'm embarrassed to say that there was actually blood drawn a couple of times, it was that bad!

Then, finally, *finally*, after close to six weeks of working with him on a daily basis, just repeatedly giving and taking away toys, treats, bones, whatever, he *finally* stopped being aggressive!

It had worked! Blessed be! Satan was gone! I had knocked the nasty out of Harold! No more Satan's child! Thank God I did, because a couple weeks later, on Halloween, my adorable great-niece Ayla, who was two years old at the time and not scared of anything, was going to put our training to the test.

Ayla had come to our house for my annual kids' Halloween party. She had found a stray bone under one of our couches. Ayla toddled over and ever so sweetly gave Harold the bone, then away she went.

However, she then decided that she wanted to go back over to Harold, who was happily chewing on the bone that she had just given him, and it turned into what I call a "slow motion movie moment." Her Grammy, my BFF Julie, and I were watching what was about to take place, but it was as though we were frozen in place. We watched little Ayla walk over, grab Harold's head, and rip that bone right out of his mouth without him so much as batting an eye at her!

Julie and I were still not breathing when Ayla turned around and did the funniest thing: she took the same bone and kept trying to shove it right back into Harold's mouth again and again. He wouldn't take it back at that point because I was watching him and I hadn't told him it was okay. What a good boy.

Thankfully I had done my due diligence with him and he was amazing with her because this could have ended very, very differently. It has always made me very proud when I hear my best friend say to people, "If Brenda says her dogs are okay around my kids, grandkids, or other kids, then they are, because I trust her training." Thanks, Jules!

Brenda Boemer-Groenestege

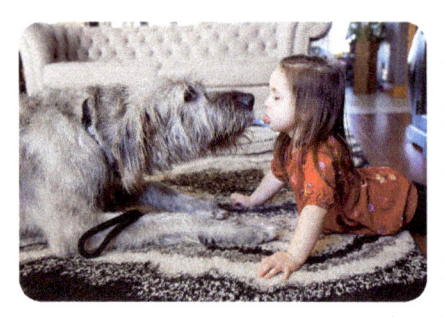

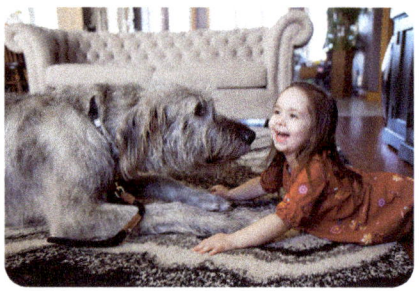

Ayla and Harold

MOVING ON WITH MORE TRAINING TECHNIQUES

When you're training your puppy, use one or two words, and, *ladies, deepen your voices* as much as you can because dogs respond best to men's voices. I call it my *demon voice*. Why is this? It quite simply goes hand in hand with vocal pitch and how dogs perceive what we are telling them or asking of them. When you speak in a low tone, it will come across more firm or cautionary to your dog which is what you want. It's not about being loud, it's completely and utterly about being obeyed. Therefore, dig deep and find the right voice that works for you and your dog when it comes to them listening and quite possibly keeping them, and you, safe.

Now is not the time to coddle your pup! If it's doing something wrong, a stern NO! Or Don't! DOWN! OFF! And of course your puppy is teething, so it's going to bite you, so you're going to say "NO BITE."

Another term I want you to learn is "Drop it" or "It's MINE." And when you're using this term, you are not using a high-pitched hyper voice, chasing your puppy around and making a game out of getting whatever your pup has! You are going to deepen your voice, say it as loud as you can, and if you can stomp your foot really hard to startle your pup, chances are he or she will drop whatever it is.

Now, after the pup drops it, do NOT praise the daylights out of the pup because obviously the pup wasn't supposed to have whatever it was in the first place. So, let's go over that again but I'm going to put it in perspective.

AN EXPLOSIVE TRUE STORY;

This is why you want to teach your dog "Drop it" or "It's Mine."

Lucky's Way

My sister Carmen and my brother-in-law Ken were having a Canada Day party. There were lots of people there: friends, family, neighbours, and kids of all sizes, from two to seventy-two. When the sun went down, Ken began to set up for fireworks.

They did everything right. They had built a large sand pit base for the fireworks and made sure it was far enough away from the house, they made sure that everyone was safely far enough away from the fireworks pit, and, most importantly, the person in charge of the fireworks was still very capable of performing their duty of setting them up and setting them off.

The one variable that Carmen and Ken didn't plan on was their big yellow Labrador Retriever, Baden. He was an awesome dog! You could throw a ball one hundred times and he would bring it back to you one hundred and one! He loved the game! He loved water and swimming, and he loved people. He was such a Lab.

Baden would frequently play in the sandbox with Carmen and Ken's kids, or try to get the kids to play with him by dropping the ball over and over again beside them, until they would get so fed up, they would hide the ball in the sand. But Baden wasn't stupid, so he would dig his ball out, and then that became a game too for a while.

So on Canada Day, while everyone was waiting for the fireworks display to start, Baden focused on one thing…what's Dad burying in the sand? And as soon as Ken lit the firecracker and ran back, Baden saw his opening, ran up to the sandbox, and grabbed the firecracker just as it was about to explode!

It was absolute chaos! Carmen was screaming (unfortunately, in a high-pitched voice, because she was, understandably, scared), Ken was yelling, everyone was yelling and trying to catch Baden!

All of a sudden, *ppppeeshhhhheeewww*, out comes the first fireball from the end of the firecracker in Baden's mouth. He still isn't dropping it, because it's a game, remember? And because everyone is running and chasing him, he's very excited and running around like crazy too. More and more fireballs come flying out, one after the other! One hit Carmen in the upper leg! Oh my gosh! That was the scariest part but Carmen didn't even care about herself, she was only worried about Baden and if he was hurt. Finally, Ken caught him, and no, Baden was not hurt.

Carmen had a huge bruise on her thigh for quite some time after that night. They never again let Baden stay outside if there was going to be fireworks going off.

I know it's very hard to stay calm in emergency situations, but if at all possible, when something like this happens, please, take a breath, remain calm, and use your demon voice. Chasing makes it a game. Hindsight is always 20/20, and easy for me to say, you may be thinking, but I'm quite sure that before something big happens, there are multiple times that something smaller happened that would have allowed you to practice this, for example, your dog took a whole cooked chicken from the counter and now doesn't want to give it up, or maybe your puppy has taken off with your new shoe, or how about when the darn dog takes off with the packaging of last night's take-out supper. Trust me when I say that things like this can happen with even the best-trained dogs on occasion…heck, my dogs do things all the time that make me shake my head and I do this for a living, for heaven's sake!

FOR THE LOVE OF…KITTENS?

It was harvest season, and I got a phone call from my son Spencer. He was pulling into our yard in the tractor and said to me very casually, "Yeah, Mom, Harold's got something in his mouth. I think it's a kitten; you might want to come outside and check."

Oh Crap! Okay, I used the other word, but I flew out of the house and yup, there's my 150-pound dog with a wee kitten hanging out of his mouth. I put my hands on my hips and growled at him "Drop it! It's mine!" Thankfully, he did, though begrudgingly.

He didn't like dropping his baby because he really does love cats, and wants his little friend back, but he doesn't realize how big he is and how dangerous it gets when his brothers are around the kitten as well. So, after drying her off, a thorough examination, and some cuddling on my part, the kitten was just fine. I gave her back to her very ticked-off mama in the barn. Harold got a stern talking to.

Lucky's Way

Harold wouldn't kill a kitten on purpose, it's just that he's got a lot of love to give and no kitten that small could handle that much love. She now lives at my neighbours' farm, much to Harold's dismay.

The moral of my story is…teach your puppy early on to "drop it"! It could save lives!

DEALING WITH THE BITING CHEWING STAGE OF PUPPYHOOD

When training your puppy, always keep your words short and to the point. "No" is probably going to be the word your puppy hears most the first weeks. I've often thought of naming my dogs that, but eventually they do start to listen. Another question I get asked all the time is about puppies biting and how to stop them from doing it. The short answer is, there is no way, not in the first couple weeks. My method is to either pull their mouth off you or flick their nose with my fingers and say "no bite" in a stern voice.

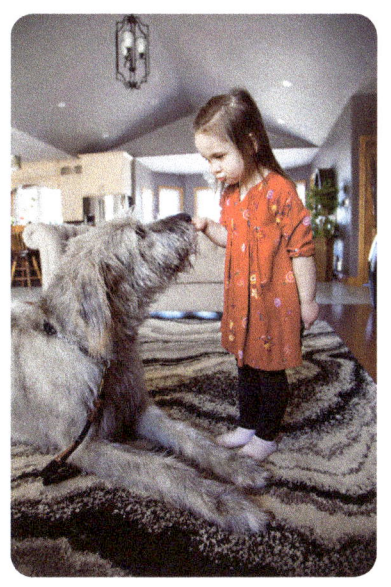

Here, Ayla is demonstrating using a firm look on Harold (holy cuteness, right?)

Having lots of dog friendly toys and chewable treats for them is also beneficial at this stage, so grab one and give one of those to them in place of your hand or your furniture. It will get monotonous, but in the end it will be for the best.

Brenda Boemer-Groenestege

LEARNING THE 10–4 RULE

There is one constant rule that applies when training your dog…repeat a command over and over again for ten minutes a day, four days in a row, without distractions, and your dog should have it ingrained in them forever. I call this the 10–4 rule.

No cell phone, no TV, no iPad, no kids, no showing off to friends while doing it, NO DISTRACTIONS! It's just you and your dog for ten minutes a day, repeating the same command over and over again for four days in a row, and he or she should have it. And praise, praise, praise after they get it! That's all your dog really wants from you anyway, lots of love.

Oh, and never leave a session on a bad note. So, if you're teaching your dog something extra difficult and it's not turning out exactly how *you* think it should be going, please don't get upset with your dog and have a human temper tantrum and stomp off. Instead, sit down, look your dog in the eye, and say to him or her, "I know this is a hard one, pal, but I know you can do it," and give your buddy a hug.

Taking a little break and making direct eye contact with your dog gives both of you a greatly needed boost. And when a dog makes eye contact with you, they are actually giving you a mental hug.

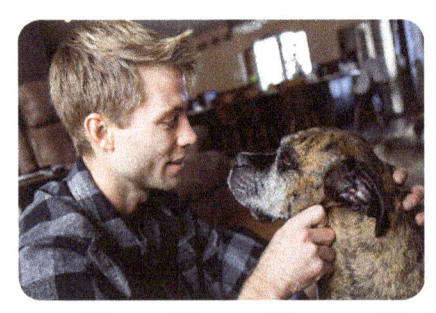

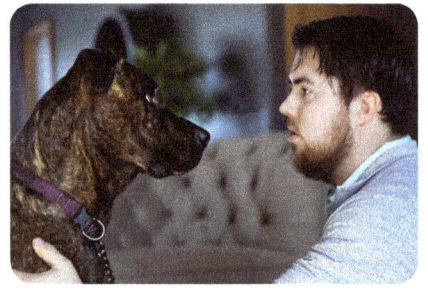

Dylan and Hogan and Spencer and Hemi, both demonstrating mental hugs perfectly.

TEACHING YOUR PUPPY TO SIT

Start with a small treat in your hand and get the attention of your pup. Then hold your hand high over and slightly behind your pup's head and say "sit." If he doesn't sit by gravity alone, push his bottom down gently with your hand, into the sitting position. When he sits, say "*good sit*" in a very happy positive voice. And, of course, give him the treat. Repeat this over and over again until your puppy goes into the "sit" position on your command immediately.

Practice this without treats as well so your puppy doesn't always expect a reward. And always finish your daily training session with your pup on a high note with lots of love and praise.

Remember to keep your focus on your dog while you work with him or her. Turn off your TV and your cell phone, ask your kids to play quietly in a different room for ten minutes. Training now means well-behaved later. Apply the 10–4 rule.

Now, the other neat little twist on my training technique is that I also use my index finger and I point at my dog and say the word sit and they sit. I've used this training method with all my dogs and I do this because it doesn't matter if you are three years old or ninety-three, you can point your finger at any one of my dogs and they will listen to your command and sit. And if you continue to point, they will lie down…at least they're supposed to!

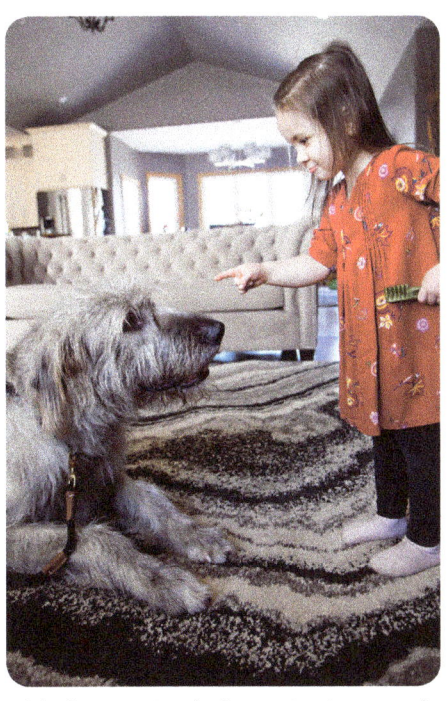

Ayla demonstrating the finger point sit command.

TEACHING PUPPY DOWN

Once your pup has mastered "sit," move on to "down." Start by asking your pup to sit, then say "down" and show him or her the treat as you bring your hand to the floor. Most dogs will automatically stand up again and just put their heads down. Say "no" and start all over again by giving him the sit command and bringing your hand to the floor again.

You may have to repeat this several times before your pup understands what you want him to do but he will figure it out. Keep practicing the sit and down and remember to give lots of praise. Don't forget the 10–4 rule.

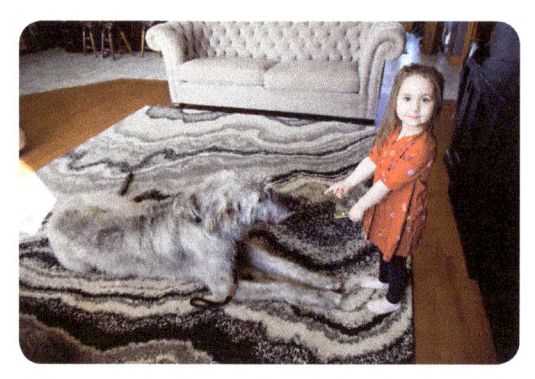

Ayla once again, showing off her skills and placing Harold in a "down" position using her finger.

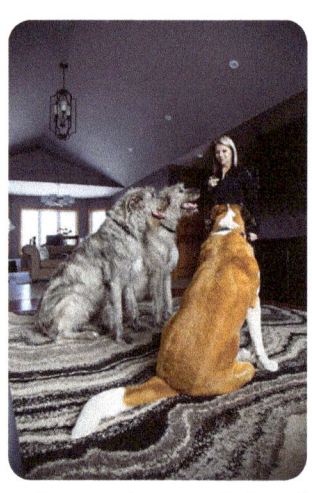

I'm not nearly as cute, but my method is still effective. Harold, Leonard, and Lloyd are with me.

TEACHING PUPPY TO STAY

Okay, I will move on to "stay." Training your dog to stay is valuable; it can save its life at some point. If, by chance, your dog has gotten loose and is running around and runs back because you called them back, and you notice a vehicle coming, you can yell "*STAY*"! All the training you put into the "stay" command when he was a pup just saved his life. So, let's get started.

Now your puppy has mastered sit and down. Once he's in the "down" position, put your hand, with the palm facing up to your pup and say, firmly, "stay," and take a step back. If your pup goes to move, say it again, keeping your hand up and still speaking firmly: "*stay*." Depending on the age of your puppy, you may only get one or two steps away from him the first day or even week of practicing "stay" command. However, as your puppy matures, you will move farther and farther away from him or her and eventually you should only have to say "stay" once.

With more practice, and the right breed of dog, you can just hold up the palm of your hand and not even use your voice. Now, here is where the 10–4 rule may not really apply. It depends on your puppy, its age, and the breed as well. So don't get discouraged if it takes more than four days to master this one.

TEACHING PUPPY TO COME

Right after "stay," of course, we move to "come." You would think this would be easy for the dog to learn but, surprisingly, it can be quite difficult, because you are essentially undoing exactly what you just taught them to do with the "stay." It can get frustratingly comical at times, but that's the beauty of working with animals.

The best way to get your pup to come to you is to bribe them—yup, I said it, bribe them. I know that goes against the "Don't use treats to train" rule, but this is a difficult command for your puppy to pick up. Yes, some puppies will be intelligent enough to get it without using treats, but mine haven't been. This method has worked for me and I stand by it, even if I'm not proud of how I get the results. Hey, if it ain't broke, don't fix it.

It's good to be organized. Make sure you have treats big enough or smelly enough to entice your pup. It should only take a few bribery-induced commands to get your dog to figure out that when you say "come" and either slap the side of your thigh or the front of your legs (whatever you choose), he pops up and runs to you to get that yummy treat. He'll have that figured out in no time. But don't forget to make him sit when he gets to you. And once again, the 10–4 rule applies here.

TEACHING YOUR PUPPY OR ADULT DOG TO TAKE TREATS POLITELY

At this point, let's take a minute to make sure your puppy is taking the treats from you gently. No one likes a nippy dog.

If your dog is a little (or a lot) too grabby when it comes to taking treats by hand, my suggestion is that you hold the treat inside the palm of your hand, keeping your fingers curled inwards, while saying to him or her, "gentle, gentle." When, and only when, your dog has stopped being super-mouthy and uses a more gentle mouth, you give him or her the treat. This is followed by "good [insert dog's name here], nice gentle gentle, good boy/girl." And once again, the 10–4 rule.

It's a joke in my family that I like to "baby bird" my dogs, which means I will take a bite of something, chew it once or twice, pry open my dog's mouth, and spit it in—yummy, right?! Okay, Okay, I'm a sick human being, but that led to me putting a treat in my lips and my dogs taking it from my lips without biting me.

Not only will my enormous 85-pound Irish Wolfhound Harold do this with me, but he does it with my four-year-old great-nephew Emmett as well and Emmett thinks it's freaking hilarious when he does it. You can see the video on my Facebook page.

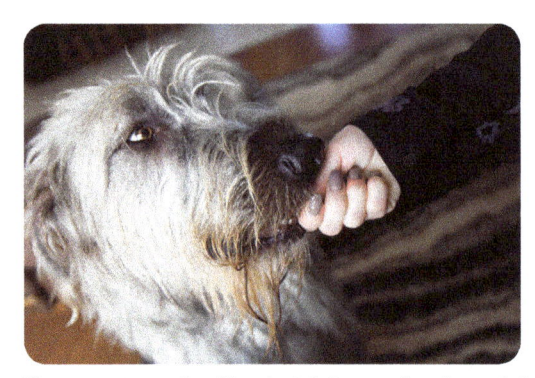

The treat is in my closed hand while I repeat "gentle, gentle."

Lucky's Way

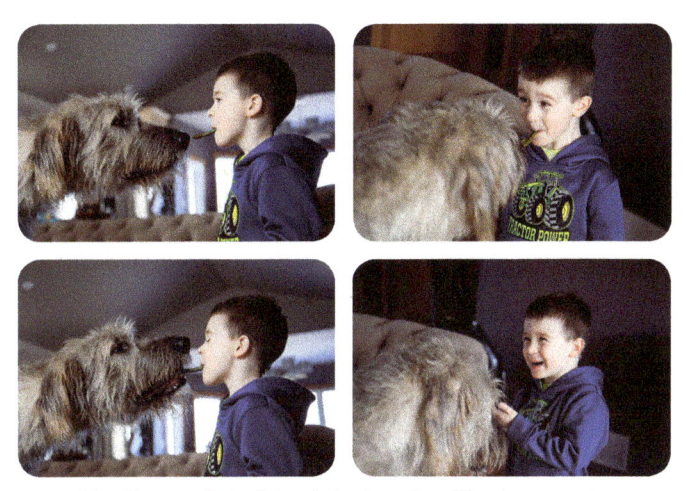

Meet Emmett...he is obviously having a lot of fun demonstrating how Harold takes treats gently from his mouth.

UNWANTED KISSING OR LICKING

On the subject of dogs' mouths, let's talk licking or "kisses" and how to keep it under control. I realize there are some people out there who don't mind the nonstop kisses that their dog gives them, but please realize that other people don't appreciate the same show of affection from your dog that you do. Therefore, if you happen to have a dog that is a licking machine, here is my quick tip to get your dog or puppy to stop.

Every time she starts licking, grab her tongue! Not hard, since you are not trying to hurt the dog, you are simply attempting to irritate her by grabbing ahold of her tongue gently. It's never about hurting your pup, only about getting their attention. This must be done consistently. If there are more people living in your house, please make sure they are all doing the same thing. The more people do it, the faster your dog will stop the behaviour.

Only after you have completely stopped this behaviour and are confident that it is something that your dog will not pick up again can you begin training your dog to give kisses on command. But *only* on your terms. You must make that clear. If you start to notice that the licking is resuming, then stop and go back to grabbing his or her tongue to once again reinforce that it is an unwanted behaviour. Unfortunately, some dogs just can't differentiate between the two, and kisses can't be given without getting out of control.

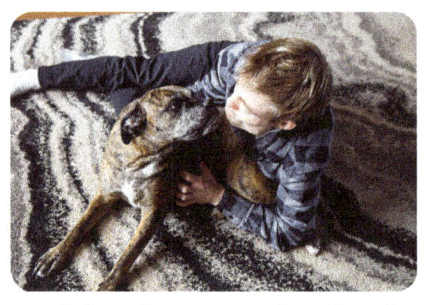

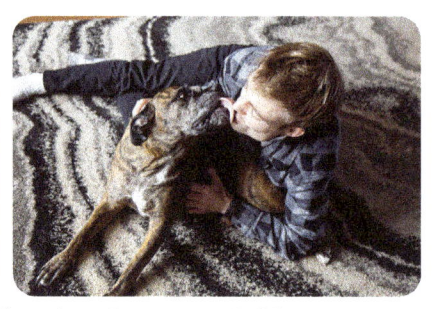

Dylan is demonstrating asking Hogan for a kiss, always being in control of the situation.

TEACH YOUR DOG TO WALK PROPERLY ON A LEASH

Teaching your dog to walk on a leash is really basic training, and should be started at an early age.

The best kind of collar to use, in my opinion, is a martingale, which is similar to a choker chain except that it is made with solid material, either leather or vinyl, and there's a portion of it that is a choker chain. You will have your puppy's martingale collar pulled up high on their neck, positioned directly behind their ears, for maximum effectiveness.

When you start your walk, your puppy or dog should always be on your *left-hand side*, right beside your thigh. Your dog's head should never be in front of you! NEVER! That means your dog is leading you, meaning it's the boss, meaning you're not, and that's not what you want! I can't stress this enough, people, you must keep your dog controlled, especially when you're first training him or her.

Teach your puppy the right way when it's young and your walks will be calm and relaxing for the life of your dog; let them have their way without proper training and you'll be stressed and hate walking your dog and have no one to blame but yourself (if you've had the dog since puppyhood).

This method works for dogs of all ages and backgrounds. Whether you adopted an adult dog, or got an eight week old puppy, collar placement and walking properly is always the same.

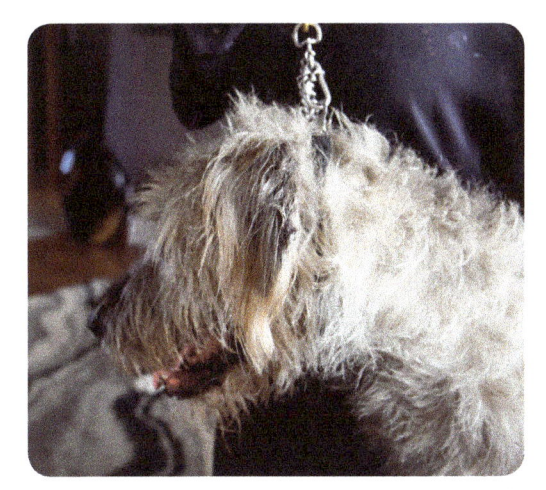

Collar placement directly behind the ears when you are walking.

Your puppy's immediate reaction will most likely be to pull back on the leash and sit down or lay down. That's completely normal; just give a gentle tug and use the command "come come" in a friendly higher-pitched tone so puppy knows he's not in trouble, and when he does start walking toward you, keep the momentum going with a quick verbal praise ("good puppy" or "good walking") and keep the leash somewhat taunt, again, always on your left side.

When you stop, puppy should stop and be trained to sit down. So, if you haven't already gotten that worked into his training, it's a quick pull up on the leash and the verbal command "sit," and if you have to, using mild pressure on his bottom, pressing down to make him sit. Practice this. When you want to start walking again, you're going to give your pup the verbal command "walk on" and then take a few steps forward, stop, verbal command "sit," and repeat. Keep doing this over and over again until your pup is confidently doing this on its own.

Now, chances are, at the beginning of your puppy's training, if you're starting right at the eight-week mark, he's going to actually get exhausted way before he picks up on the exercise. Don't sweat it. Just keep trying. Keep in mind that a tired puppy means a good night's sleep for human parents.

As your pup grows and learns, keep adding to their training. After they have basic leash-walking and "stop," "sit," "down" skills, you can start to train them to ignore people and other dogs or distractions around them.

Another part of walking your dog is your own body language. Be sure that you yourself remain confident when you're walking, and always look straight ahead. Anticipate obstacles before your dog sees them so you know ahead of time what you may need to address. Showing your dog that you are confident will help them relax and enjoy their walk and lessen their need to think they have to protect you.

Generally speaking, misbehaved dogs take their cues from their owners. The owner sees other dogs coming and right away begins to get anxious; your dog feels that tension and anxiety and automatically goes into defensive mode, thinking they have to protect you. Instead, square your shoulders, stand tall, and walk with purpose. If your dog even remotely starts to react to the oncoming dog, person, or whatever, you immediately jerk his leash, which will snap his collar, and give him a little right-foot back-flank kick action that should distract him enough to continue on.

In the case of some of my giant breed friends, poke them in the shoulder…you'll get the same result. It's a distraction, a momentary attention disruption.

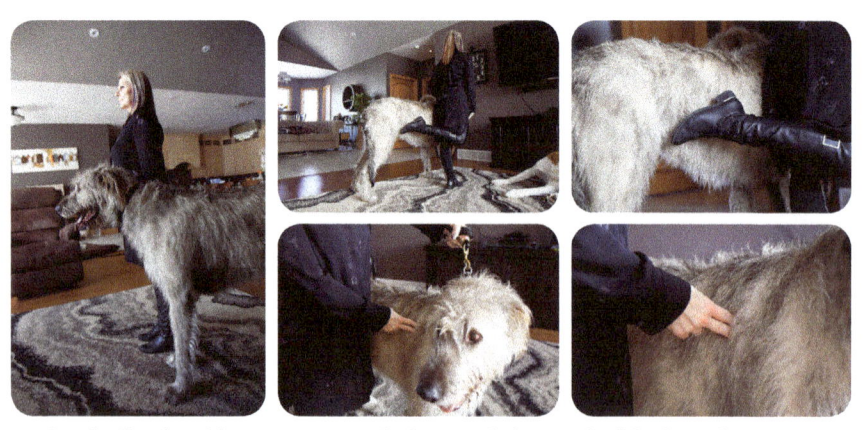

Stand tall and confident. Using your right foot, tap the hip or side of the dog to distract him. Poking him in the shoulder will get the same result.

Can dogs suffer from ADHD? Hyperactivity, also known as hyperkinesis, are dogs who display frenetic activity, extremely short attention spans and a high impulsiveness to react to something that catches their attention… it is truly a canine form of Attention Deficit Hyper-Activity Disorder (ADHD). If you don't think your dog suffers from this, have them focus on a toy and then have someone walk in the room; I guarantee your dog will breaks the stare from the toy and look to the person even just for a second. Then they see a squirrel outside, or, a shiny object!

That's my grand-dog Hogan's weakness: anything shiny and she's on it! A reflection, a laser, a flashlight.

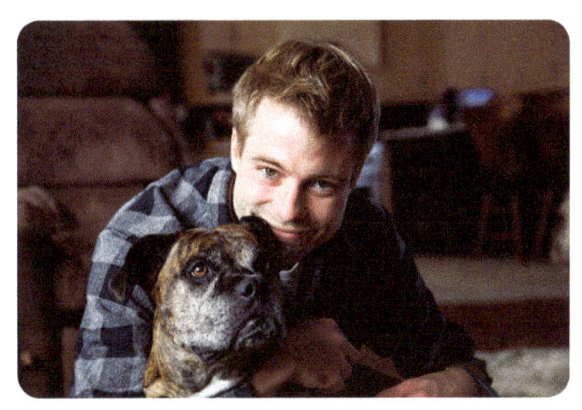

Dylan and his dog, Hogan (she is a mix of boxer, American bulldog, and American mastiff). She's incredibly smart and Dylan does everything with her, including paddle boarding (FYI; always make sure you fit your dog properly with a canine life vest when spending time on the water with them - even though all dogs know how to swim instinctively, there can always be mitigating factors that could cause your dog to drown, therefore, better safe than sorry).

TEACHING THE COMMAND "HOT"!
Now, this may not seem very important when you are first skimming through this book, but, trust me, this is a very important lesson to teach your dog, especially if you have a dog that can reach the height of your oven.

Whenever I open my oven door and one of my dogs is around, I say "Watch—Hot" in a cautious tone. So, let's cover that tone—it's not the singsong happy voice we use when puppy does something good and it's not the deep "hell hath no fury" voice that we use when we are demanding that our rotten dog drop the pork chop he just stole from the counter.

When I'm drinking my tea and my dog wants to smell or lick my teacup, I say "Hot," in that cautious tone. It works great if you're into sharing food with your dog and it's hot. Just like with a child, you say, "Oh, it's hot" and blow on it and then share it with your dog.

Harold, he's my big boy Wolfhound and by far my biggest pain in the butt while I'm cooking. He's always nosing around the island and the stove and no matter how many times I give that big thug heck, he's right there, literally in my face, sniffing the air, or almost getting his nose chopped off when I'm chopping away on the island, just waiting for me to drop a morsel of food for him! Anything: a crumb, peeling, a crust, he doesn't care as long as he gets it before one of his brothers does.

Now, for those of you who have a giant breed dog, the other danger in your kitchen is your stove. Gas or electric, both could be catastrophic. I love to cook so I have a big six-burner gas stove that I adore, but when Harold brings over that big gorgeous hairy head of his and I see it inch closer and closer to the gas flame of my stove…well, holy spicy meatballs, my heart damn near stops!

So, what do I do? Well, I take a page out of my daughter, Brooklyn's, "how to annoy the crap out of your dog" handbook (*not a real book btw), and I grab my stainless steel tongs and snap them in his face and say "Back—Hot—Owie!" This seems to work! Thank goodness for stainless steel tongs and Brooklyn!

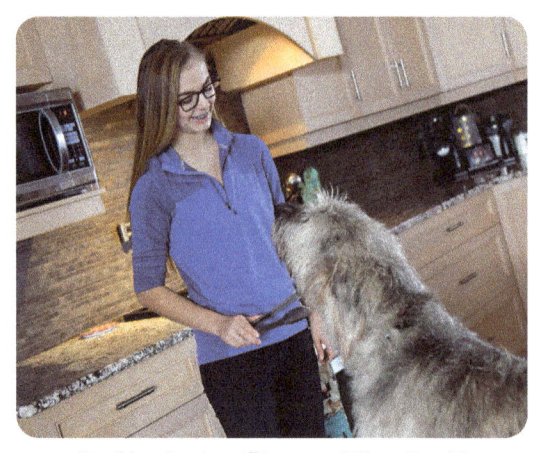

Brooklyn showing off her tong skills to Harold.

DEALING WITH AGGRESSION

This is a very challenging subject to address and a difficult issue to go through with your dog. It doesn't matter if your dog is 10 lb, 110 lb, or 210 lb, you must get an aggressive dog in check and keep it that way!

First, you have to determine what's causing the aggressive behaviour. Is it insecurity? Did something happen to bring it on? Is your dog trying to protect you? Is your dog just simply aggressive by nature? Chances are it's one of the first two and there's an even bigger chance that you are feeding into your dog's aggression unknowingly.

When dealing with aggression, you have to determine the root cause. Is it insecurity in the dog or is he actually feeling that he has to protect you or a family member or someone or something in his surroundings?

To stop this behaviour, you have to catch it just as the dog is beginning the poor behaviour. When you see your dog about to start to growl or bark, that's when you make your move. You need to snap him out of it by getting his attention and changing his focus from whatever he was turning his aggression on back to you.

Now, how do we do this? It's really quite easy. Just before he starts this bad behaviour and you notice that he's going to growl or become aggressive, you tap him on the side or on the shoulder or give him a quick shove in the hip (whatever works, whatever will get his attention off what he's focused on and onto you) and you say to him, "No." I use the catchphrase, "Mind your business" or "That's not your business."

When I'm walking four giant breed dogs, I cannot have one of them focused on, or becoming aggressive, toward an oncoming dog being walked by a person who doesn't have their dog under control. Leonard just recently stopped doing that. I'm not sure if it was a little bit of insecurity or if he felt that he was protecting me; either way it is unacceptable behaviour.

The worst possible reaction is to pet your dog while it's barking and growling and say, "It's okay, it's okay, it'll be fine, don't do that," because what you're doing is condoning the behaviour. You're actually encouraging your dog to growl and become more aggressive because he thinks that he's doing a good job. Your dog believes that you're petting him in encouragement; he will continue to be aggressive, and this reaction will just escalate his aggression.

You must be the dominant pack leader. You need to show your dog that you *do not* need him to stand up for you. The only way to do this is for you to be the boss. The minute your dog starts to become aggressive, you have to take charge of the situation and stop the behaviour.

Reading the situation before anything even happens is the best way to keep it under control. If you're out for a walk and you see another dog or person approaching and you know your dog is going to react, you immediately say to your dog, "mind your business" or "behave" or whatever your catchphrase is, so your dog knows that you **do not** need him or her to protect you.

When you have been dealing with an aggressive dog for a while, you may become so nervous and so afraid that the energy you're giving off feeds into your dog's negative behaviour. It becomes a vicious cycle. The more you stress, the more your dog is going to react to your insecurities and behave accordingly.

Now, how do you overcome your own fears and insecurities when it comes to your dog's aggression? YOU MUST BE CONFIDENT! Only you can rectify your dog's behaviour, because he or she is feeding off you. When you prove that you do not need your dog to stick up for you, then your dog will stop the behaviour. Let's break it down.

First and foremost:

- BE CONFIDENT—showing confidence reinforces that you are the alpha!

- Use the right equipment. Use a proper collar, such as a Herm Sprenger martingale collar for a particularly large, strong breed, or just a martingale collar for any other size and breed of dog, and make sure you have it positioned high up on his or her neck, right behind the ears, so you have control of his or her head. (See picture under "Learning to walk on a leash")

- Taking stock of your surroundings is key to being confident with your dog. Anticipating your dog's triggers before he or she does removes the need for them to react negatively. You have already

Lucky's Way

shown them that you've got the situation under control and therefore they have nothing to react to.

- When they spot the trigger, quickly and confidently pull up on the collar and simultaneously tap their hind end with your right foot, thus changing their focus back to you. They're going to look at you like, "What? Why'd you kick me?" You are simply rerouting their focus from what would normally trigger them to react negatively to simply reacting by focusing on you.

- When you remain calm, cool, and collected, and prove that you DO NOT need them for protection, they will stop the behaviour, and both you and your dog will enjoy your walks.

- Remember, practice makes perfect!

This is something that has to be addressed over and over again, repeatedly, until the aggression is completely gone from the dog and the dog knows that that particular behaviour is no longer going to be tolerated and that there's no reason for it.

Determining whether your dog is being aggressive because of insecurity or whether your dog is being aggressive because it's being protective is not always easy.

Having your dog bark when people come to the door isn't the worst thing in the world, at least in my opinion. But you need to be able to step up and say to your dog, "That's enough. Sit" and have them settle down and not attack whoever is on the other side of your door.

We live on a hundred-acre farm and I'll admit that I feel a lot more comfortable knowing that when people pull in our driveway, they're a little hesitant getting out of their vehicle not only because of the size of our dogs, but because a couple of them are barking and causing a fuss. That's perfectly okay with me because that's their job.

However, when I give them the command "That's enough" and call them off, they must listen to me, come to the house, and know that I have the situation under control.

There have been times when a strange vehicle (even to me) pulls in, and I have attempted to call the dogs off and they have not listened to me. That's when I think to myself, hey, maybe I should be extra careful here, because the dogs have a sixth sense, and I go with it, because, quite often, they know better than I do.

There are times when it is better to contact a professional dog handler and ask for their help in assessing your dog's aggressive behaviour. If you feel that you are unable or ill-equipped to deal with the situation on your own, then I urge you to seek the advice of a professional dog trainer.

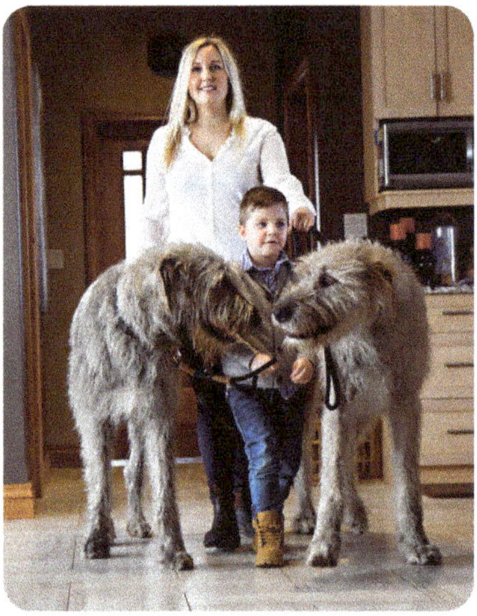

Picture 1 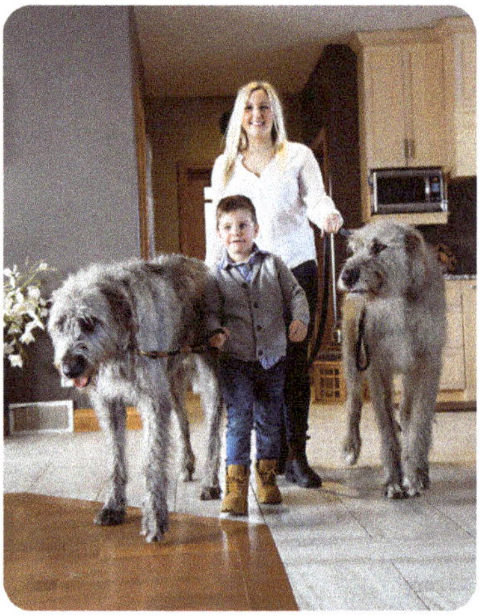 *Picture 2*

These pictures are a perfect example of dominance through looks.

Picture 1 shows Harold glaring at Leonard and picture 2 shows Leonard backing away. We had no idea that this happened until we were reviewing the pictures and I got a good look at them, but you can clearly see the look in Harold's eyes. Harold is "claiming" that Lincoln and Jody are his and Leonard needs to back off, and it is very clear that Harold is the alpha dog, therefore Leonard does what is expected of the omega dog.

CHAPTER 7

Train Your Dog to Become a Therapy Dog

If you have decided to train your dog as a therapy dog, the training starts the day you pick up your puppy. What's the difference between training a therapy dog and a regular family pet? Well, you must be a lot more strict when it comes to things your pup is and is not allowed to do, and you have to start exposing your dog to EVERYTHING!

I can't stress this enough. Get yourself a training vest for your dog that says "Therapy Dog In Training" and bring him or her with you wherever you go. (You can find these vests at Service Dogs Canada, https://www.servicedogscanada.org.) This is done after you've completed proper early training with your puppy and are confident that there won't be any accidents while in a store or indoor area.

Your dog should be well-behaved, friendly, confident, calm, and well socialized. He should be able to hold his natural urges until you deem fit to take him outside. Yes, this sounds harsh, but it is necessary for a therapy dog. I started getting my dogs to "hold in" their natural urges by making them hold off at home when they'd go to the door and I knew they wanted out to go to the bathroom. I would say to them, "No, you have to hold it." I would then make them wait 5–30 minutes, depending on their age, and then I would take them out and say "Go pee pee" and of course they would go right away. Now, mind you, if they are standing at the door and whining their poor little head off, then I knew it was bad and they needed to go immediately and I would never ever make them hold it in.

So now, when we are out for therapy, one session usually runs approximately one hour before we take a break; if one of my boys goes to the door and scratches it, I just say those magic words "No, you have to hold it," and they'll come back to the group and continue to participate. On occasion, the puppy still needs to go out during therapy, which is quite normal since he's just four months old at the time of me writing this book and therefore his holding ability isn't where his older brothers' are yet.

Just one more thing about bathroom breaks and then we'll move on, I promise! I prefer my male dogs to pee like females. This does not emasculate them by any means; what it does is prevent them from peeing on everyone's trees from here to Timbuktu! How can you accomplish this, you ask? Well, you keep your male dog on a leash and don't encourage him to pee on trees, posts, plants, steps, etc. Just let them urinate on the grass.

Moving on, taking your puppy into public is a great way to start to expose them to the therapy world. The more people and situations the better. Get them use to strange noises and sounds such as buses and trucks, fire trucks and police cars, and ambulances.

I'm lucky to have a nephew who is a fireman; when he's on duty, he'll actually bring the truck to my house and light it up with all the sirens going, which is great for my dogs…not so much for my neighbours, though.

It's great to take them out to the Canada Day parade. Between the bands, the clowns, the mini cars driven by the War Amps, the horses, the antique tractors, and more, the diversity of sights, sounds and smells are the perfect combination for training your therapy dog.

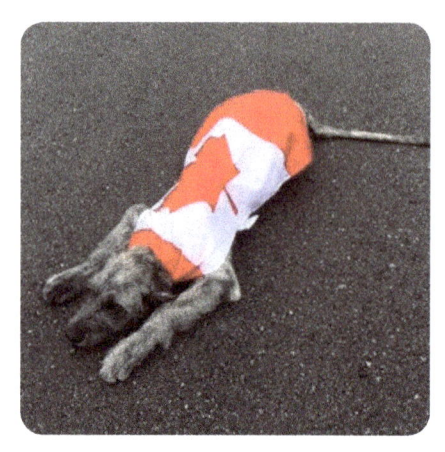

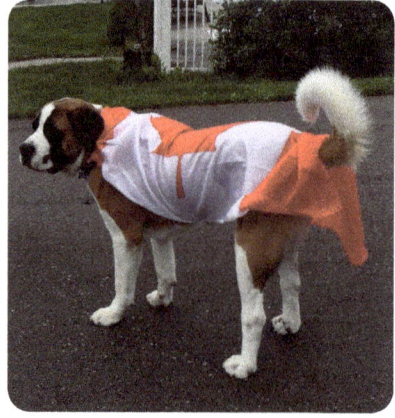

Lucky's Way

Getting your dog used to going in and out of sliding doors, or revolving doors, is a bit of a challenge. As well, the elevator comes into play in a lot of places we go. Harold is pro at the elevator. He'll actually find it and bump the buttons because he knows them so well.

Next comes training your dog to behave accordingly while at therapy. This is where the accumulation of all the months of your hard work should begin to pay off. While at therapy, your dog should behave like a champ while around other people. He or she should be calm, patient, accepting of people's affection, quiet and respectful. Not all dogs are created equal when it comes to being therapy dogs. Harold has come by it very naturally. Leonard…not so much. Does that make Leonard any less of a therapy dog than Harold? No, it just means that where Harold is strong, Leonard sits back, and where Leonard shines, Harold takes that step back.

Leonard is, by nature, a bit more timid than Harold. Therefore, he tends to be more of a follower than a leader. He's unbelievably sweet-natured when we're out on therapy duty, but at home he can be quite loud and even an aggressive guard dog, surprisingly enough. But when the vest goes on, they're on duty and they know it.

Lloyd has the same personality as Leonard; he's quite a guard dog at home, but he's a sweet-natured, loving therapy dog when we're out on the dog therapy trail.

Then there's Clark Griswald…he's definitely more like Harold. He's a natural-born therapy dog. He loves everyone and everyone loves him. And man, does he have a lot of love to give!

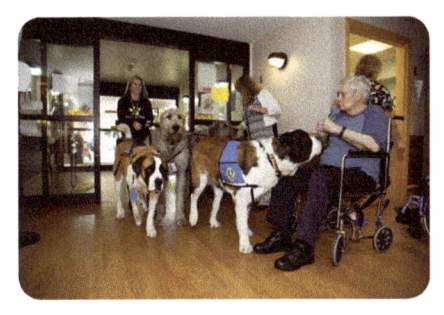

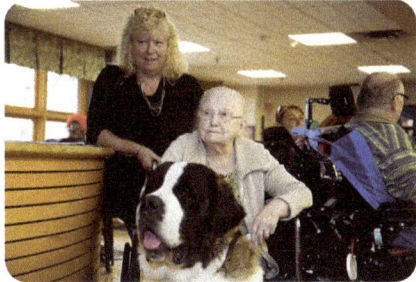

117

Brenda Boemer-Groenestege

TRAINING AN OLDER FARM DOG FOR THERAPY: IS THIS POSSIBLE?

My cousin Tanya called me to ask this question: "Is it even possible to train an older dog? My dog is just over a year old and we can't seem to get him to retain any training we've tried. I seriously think we got a defective dog!"

I had to laugh at her, because I can picture in my mind exactly what is happening at her extremely busy household. Their chocolate Lab, Jaguar, is proving to be quite the handful, so I tried to ease Tanya's mind by telling her about another chocolate Lab I worked with in early spring 2017.

I received an email from a young lady asking for help training her four-year-old chocolate Lab, Temo. He was a farm dog and therefore not used to being tied up, or leash-walked, for that matter. I asked her what her ultimate goal was for her and Temo and she told me that since she works in a nursing home, she would really love to be able to bring him in and use him as a therapy dog.

Thankfully, I was already sitting down when she told me this. Holy barking bananas! Let me get this straight…Temo is an untrained four-year-old Lab, a farm dog, who doesn't leash-walk well and doesn't live with her, he lives on the farm and she lives in the city, but she wants him trained as a therapy dog? Is this even possible? I guess we won't know unless we try, right?

Well, guess what? After some really intensive training, and a lot of hard work on the part of Temo's owner, he's doing amazing work sharing his beautiful friendly disposition with all the lovely people in the nursing home where she works. I couldn't be more proud of Temo's owner. I give her full credit. She did all the homework, and she's rockin' being the proud owner of a well-behaved, well-trained dog.

So, to answer my cousin's question…yes, Tanya, it is possible to train an older dog. You just have to be willing to put in the hard work. I think the hardest part is getting the *whole family* on board to do the same training and hard work to achieve the ultimate goal of a well-trained dog.

I see this so often. If it's one person, one dog, the training is no problem because you have no one else to blame but yourself. But when I'm working

Lucky's Way

with a family and trying to get the entire family doing the exact same techniques, that's where the challenges lie.

It's almost better if it is only one person in the family that takes on the task of training the dog initially. Then, after the dog is already trained, that one family member can train the rest of the family, who can then join in the training. Does that make sense? Clear as mud, right?

When it comes to the therapy, my boys give to others… I really can't take credit for any of it, because they do all the hard work. I'm just their chauffeur, really.

They love helping in the stroke unit and visiting in the mental health ward, and of course the nursing staff at the Stratford General Hospital always look forward to our visits because, as we all know, nurses and all hospital staff are overworked and under-appreciated.

I can go on and on about my boys and how much joy and love they bring.

One thing I love about my job is watching the before and after of our visits. I've witnessed people who are seriously stressed out walk over and completely give themselves, and their stress, to the dogs, and soon they are feeling much better. It brings me so much joy to watch this transformation.

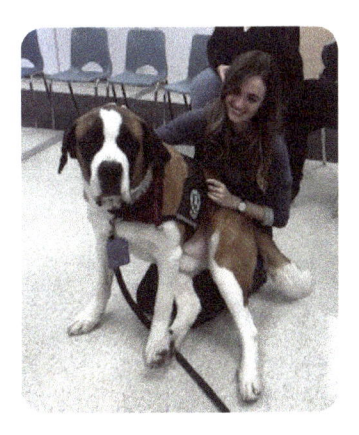

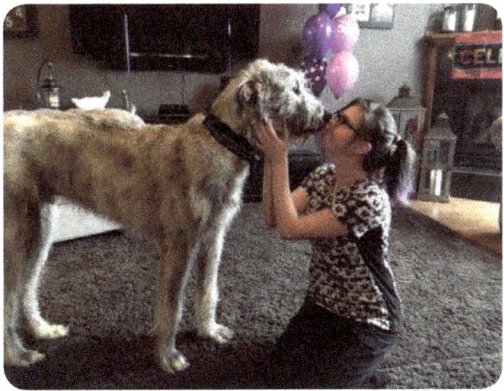

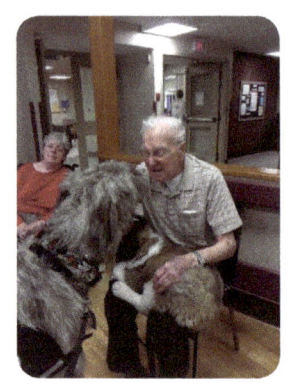

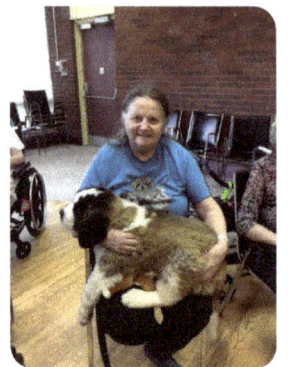

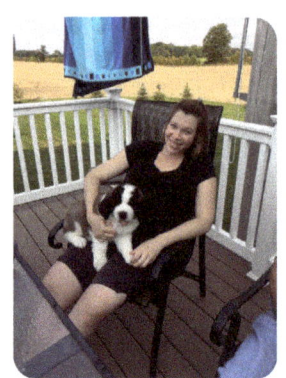

Walter, Susan and Jessica are all enjoying cuddling with Clark Griswald while he could still sit on their laps.

No matter how young or old, stressed out, upset, or sick people are, my dogs absorb every ounce of their negative energy and leave them feeling better. We have never left anyone without a smile on their face.

The great part about it is that my boys don't take their work home with them. They don't go home upset about what we saw or heard, they don't ever complain about the amount of people who hugged them or cried into their necks that day. They still come home as happy as they always are, ready to give out more love to whoever needs it at home.

I love my job!

CHAPTER 8

Frequently Asked Questions

WHAT'S THE RIGHT AGE TO GET MY DOG SPAYED OR NEUTERED?

There are so many different arguments out there when it comes to whether or not you should get your dog fixed. Here's my ten-cents worth.

In most breeds, spaying or neutering should be done around the age of six months. It's important to spay the female dog before she comes into her first heat cycle, which can be anywhere around or after the age of eight months.

In the giant breeds, however, it is my belief, and that of my father (and yes, I've done quite a bit of research on this subject as well), that unless there is a necessity for getting my dogs fixed before the age of eighteen months to two years old, I prefer to leave them intact to that age to give them the best chance of maximum growth. The disadvantage of waiting this long is that the cost is considerably more than it would have been if I had gotten them fixed at six months, because it's based on weight.

Either way, it is very important to spay or neuter your dog. Studies show that dogs who are left intact are at higher risk of cancer than those who have been fixed.

THE BENEFITS OF GASTROPEXY
(Should this be something you should consider for your dog?)
At the same time that my guys are getting fixed, I get their stomachs tacked, which is called gastropexy. Again, this is just my ten-cents worth. What exactly is a gastropexy and why did my dogs need it?

Well, a gastropexy is a procedure that permanently attaches the dog's stomach to the abdominal wall to prevent the stomach from twisting and causing GDV (Gastric Dilatation and Volvulus), also known as "bloat." Bloat is a bizarre, unpredictable, and potentially deadly condition where gas accumulates in the dog's stomach and causes the organ to twist. Left untreated, it can kill a dog within a matter of hours.

This tends to happen in the larger, deep-chested dog breeds but can occur in any breed or age of dog.

Coincidentally, while on a camping trip just a few weeks after Clark's surgery for neutering and gastropexy, we met a female Saint Bernard who had just had to have emergency gastropexy surgery done because her stomach had twisted after eating and drinking and she had literally been in the process of dying from "bloat". That surgery had cost them $4000!!! However, by choosing to have this procedure done at the same time as when your dog would be in getting spayed or neutered. In this case, this would have never happened, saving you or them quite literally thousands of dollars.

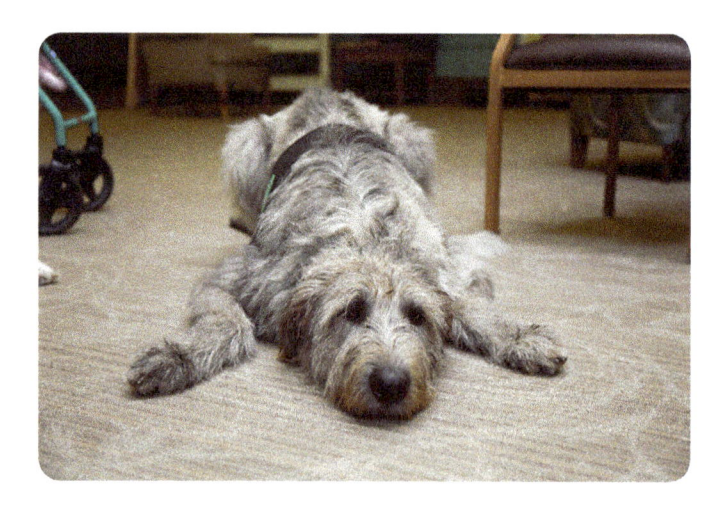

LEONARD'S STORY

Leonard was one of only two in a litter, which is unusual. From very early on, Leonard grew quickly (his nickname at the breeder was Fat Bastard, haha), and we knew he was going to be stockier than Harold because of his parents. Leonard and Harold have the same dad but different moms and Leonard's mom is considerably thicker than Harold's.

Anyhow, we noticed that Leonard was never as graceful as Harold. When he went from a lying down position to standing up, he seemed like an old man.

By the time he was approximately nine months old, I noticed that he had started limping on his hind end, so I took him to my vet and my vet noticed that Leonard had a sore toe, so we treated that with antibiotics to see if it would stop the limp. It did not. He then put Leonard on a strict regimen of rest, anti-inflammatories, and pain medication for ten days to see if that would help. Again, no difference.

Then came the "incident." It was the day before I returned home from a trip to Germany. Apparently, the dogs were all outside with Bob, and Harold was running the laps that he does around our yard when he ran, full-on, full-tilt, right into Leonard's sore leg! Bob said poor Leonard went down hard and stayed down. Bob ran over and helped Leonard up and it took quite a while before Leonard would put any weight on his leg again.

I got home the next night and heard the story. By then, Leonard seemed okay, but I booked an appointment for the following day for x-rays.

To say I was worried would be an understatement. I had no idea what we were going to find. Already, at a previous appointment, Dr. Glen had done one of the reflex tests, where you pick up your dog's foot, pull it back, and see if it springs back, naturally landing in place in its usual position. If it doesn't, like if it lands on its toes, it's bad news…well, Leonard's landed on his toes when he did it on his right hind leg.

So, when the x-ray came back and there were no fractures or cracks, that was good news, but it looked like the hip was not sitting in the socket properly, and there was also something else that I saw on the x-ray. I joked to Dr. Angela, "Oh look, he's having a baby." It was a cryptorchidism, approximately 2.5 inches long (an undescended testicle).

The prognosis at that time was that Leonard had early onset hip dysplasia and the remedy moving forward was to keep him on anti-inflammatories and try to keep him quiet. I'm a big believer in supplements, so I researched and found the best ones I could get my hands on and started him on them. Lots of glucosamine, cartilage, MSM, chondroitin, antioxidants, and more. It was a daily regime of trying to keep him quiet, giving him his meds, and keeping Leonard and Harold separated outside because, for some reason, they just weren't getting along.

Within two weeks, Harold's aggression had escalated to a level that scared not only me, but upset the whole family. We couldn't put Harold and Leonard outside together because Harold was attacking Leonard. Even indoors they started at each other.

I'd had enough. I called my vet. And I learned that the undescended testicle could be giving off female pheromones, which would be driving Harold cuckoo! Yes, that's a technical term.

I started becoming aware of how Leonard was acting toward Harold, and it was obvious that he was a very confused eleven-month-old puppy dog. Oh my! To witness, my very large 140-pound very male Irish Wolfhound prancing around, rubbing his butt in his brother's face, acting like, well, quite honestly, he was acting like a bitch in heat, and it was really, really ticking Harold off! And confusing the hell out of poor Leonard, because he had no idea what was wrong with him and why he was feeling the way he was feeling.

Harold knew his brother was male! VERY male, and it was really, really upsetting him! To the point that we could no longer allow the two of them to be alone together or Harold would unfortunately lash out at Leonard for acting the way he was.

Thankfully, we only had to wait a week before Harold went in for his surgery, but Leonard had two weeks to wait for his, so he continued on his daily quest of trying, without success, to attract a mate!

Finally, came the day of Leonard's surgery. The joke was, if it was going to go wrong, it will with Leonard, because that's just the way it was. Right from the start, Dr. Angela said that in ninety percent of dogs with cryptorchidism, it will be on the right side. With Leonard, it was on his left side. Thankfully, they had the x-ray pictures to consult to find it. Well, now they came in darn handy because between the x-ray pictures and the ultrasound, they knew exactly where to find his nugget and went in to get it. And this is where it gets interesting.

After a three-hour surgery, Dr. Angela came out to tell me that Leonard's undescended testicle had "testicular torsion," which is a condition where the spermatic cord twists around the testicle, cutting off all the blood supply as well as the elimination of metabolic waste products such as lactic acid and carbon dioxide. Ultimately, the testis becomes starved of oxygen, blood, and life-giving nutrients. So, what happens is that initially the testis becomes very swollen and enlarged and painful and then eventually it begins to die and rot within the animal.

When Dr. Angela showed me the removed testis, it was no bigger than a pecan in a shell. I was shocked, considering how large it had appeared on the x-ray just weeks before.

After we got back home and I got Leonard comfortable, I googled everything that Dr. Angela had told me and it all started making sense. Want to guess what one of the side effects of cryptorchidism is? Feminizing syndrome!

And there's more…way more! His surgery was Wednesday; I'm writing this on Sunday night…remember his limping? **NO MORE LIMPING!** We started noticing almost right away that he seemed happier. Even though the poor bugger has three incisions.

He's walking smoother, stretching out like he's never done before, AND when I pick up his back foot and drop it…it falls down perfectly! I'm telling you, I've been crying so many times over the past couple of days because I'm so happy for my sweet boy. I was so afraid that he was going to go through life in pain with arthritis or hip dysplasia and to find out that he's now, quite possibly, going to be just fine, is such a huge relief.

Of course, I will be continuing on with the supplements for him and all my dogs, as well as regular acupuncture, because I believe that gives them the best quality of life.

I want to thank the online Pet Informed site for their very informative page. I got a lot of my information from that page and I encourage anyone needing more information about this subject to look it up on their website: www.pet-informed-veterinary-advice-online.com.

Leonard is two years old and he's an incredibly happy boy. He doesn't limp at all any more, and he acts like a puppy all the time. He runs laps around the house, which is so fun to watch simply because it's something he never did before.

Brenda Boemer-Groenestege

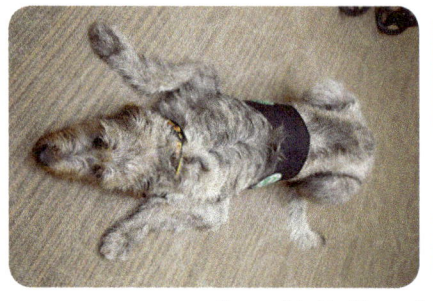

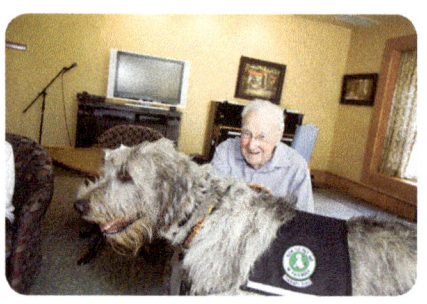

Leonard in his "frogger" pose   Leonard with Walter

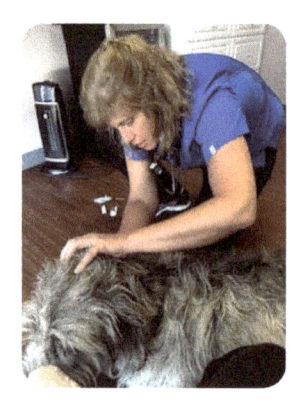

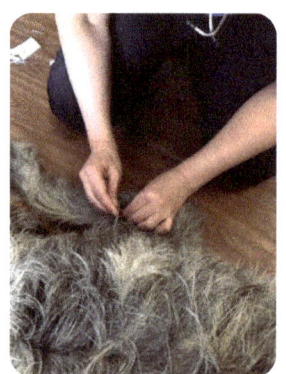

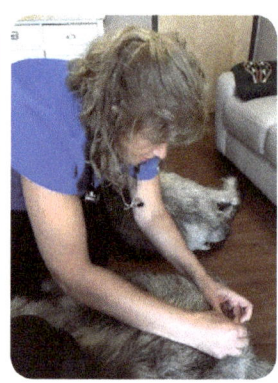

Leonard and Harold are both enjoying their acupuncture therapy from Dr. Angela

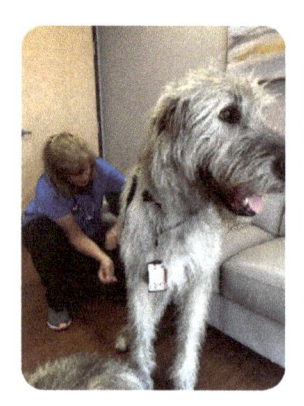

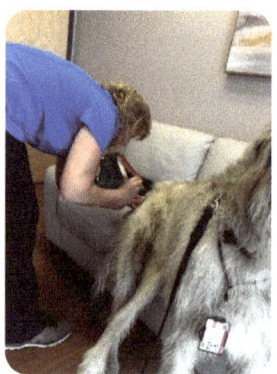

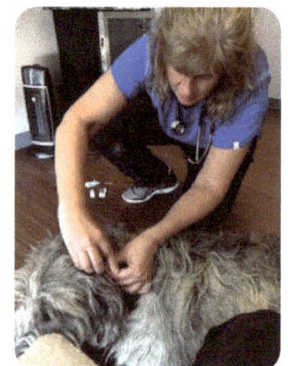

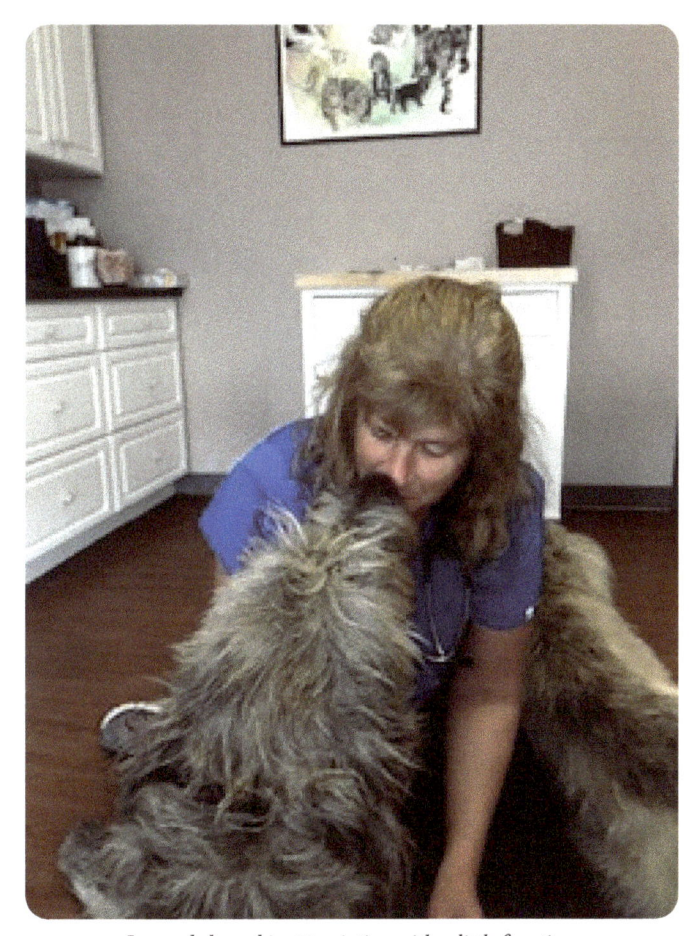

Leonard shows his appreciation with a little face time.

HOW DO I GET MY DOGS TO BEHAVE ON A WALK WHEN OTHER DOGS ARE AROUND?

This is, by far, the question that I get asked the most. These situations happen to me as well, by the way, when other people's dogs misbehave and then my dog or dogs react accordingly.

Well, here's my answer: you can only control your own reaction and that of your dog. Now, if you happen to be like me, an almost 5'3" fifty-two-year-old woman walking three or four dogs that weigh, collectively, close to seven hundred pounds, the very first things you need are *Herm Sprenger collars*… and a lot of attitude!

Brenda Boemer-Groenestege

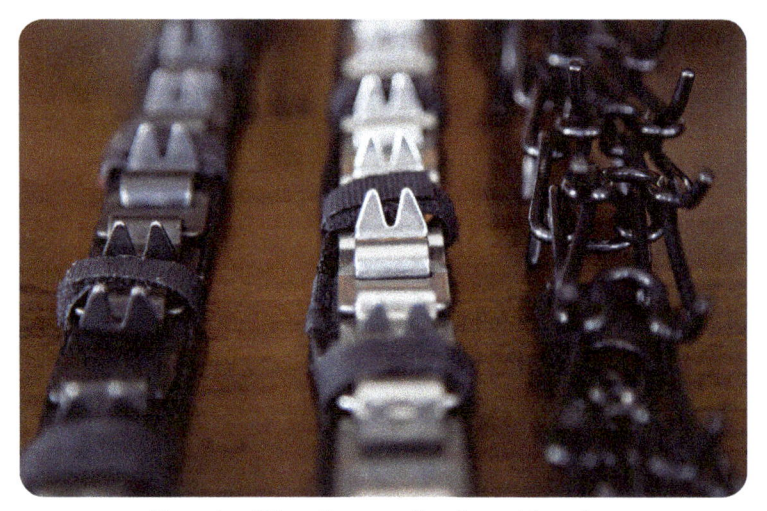

*Two styles of Herm Sprenger collars I use with my dogs.
The long prong I use on my a**hole dog, mostly because of his long hair and thick skin.*

These collars are like a-prong collars only with short v-shaped metal teeth (to mimic the teeth of a mother dog). I also have the nylon covering, so it doesn't look menacing, but one sturdy tug on this and man, do my boys pay attention. I actually call it the "a-hole" collar, because it stops them from being a-holes. I got the martingale type, which works great.

The other trick I use is the back kick. So, we're walking along and here comes a dog and my boys are paying too much attention to that dog, so I jerk their a-hole collar, tell them to "mind their own business," and swing my foot behind me and kick them in the flank or butt, just hard enough to change their focus back to me.

Another little tip I learned from watching a man named César Millán (you may have heard of him): I never stop moving forward with my dogs when other dogs are approaching. I keep walking and telling them to mind their own business, always saying "walking, boys, let's go, come on," so they know that I'm in charge of the situation and all is good and I won't tolerate any bad behaviour.

Remember, *stand tall and be confident* because your dog is feeding off your energy. See pictures on page 108.

CAN MY THREE-YEAR-OLD WALK MY GIANT BREED DOG?

This is another question I was asked regarding walking giant breeds and young children…like, really young…the exact question was "How can I train my giant breed dog to be so well-behaved on a leash that my three-year-old can walk them?"

To me, it is common sense that unless you are walking a geriatric giant breed dog, you would not let a three-year-old leash-walk a dog. *Big sigh…* here is my real answer: training your dog to walk on a leash is a must, training that same dog to be walked by a three-year-old on a leash is just plain irresponsible, for the simple reason that the minute that dog catches wind of another dog or animal that they deem may be a threat to your child, well, bye bye dog with child in tow.

Please understand that I'm being honest here, and as much as you and I want our giant breed dogs to be super-gentle all the time, their natural instinct is to protect and it will kick in one hundred percent of the time when it comes to their humans, especially their little ones.

And again, your dog may be the best-trained dog in the world, but it only takes one aggressive dog from across the street to lunge out at "Junior" while walking and your dog will protect your child without considering that they may be dragging your kid into traffic while doing so!

So what's the solution? There are two ways that your child can leash-walk your dog. First, in an enclosed backyard or secured fenced-in area. Put the leash on and let Junior walk the dog until their little legs give out. I do this with a lot of the little people in my life. I always get them to walk my Irish Wolfhounds around on the leash and tell the little kids that *they* are the boss of the dog and that *they* are in charge and therefore, if the dog isn't doing what they want, the kid has to be confident, and bossy! It's the funniest thing to watch.

The children will yell at me and say, *"The dogs aren't listening!"* And I'll yell back, *"Who is the boss?"* and the children get frustrated, puff out their chests, and square off with a dog that is quite literally five times their size and yell at them, *"I'm the boss! Let's go!"* And low and behold, the dog listens, and off they go. This is teaching children, from a very young age, to be confident, self-assured, and dominant around dogs.

Second, there are leashes that have two sets of hand loops on them. One is right down by the collar and the other is at the end of the leash. Let Junior hold the loop by the collar and you keep a firm grip on the loop on the end of the leash.

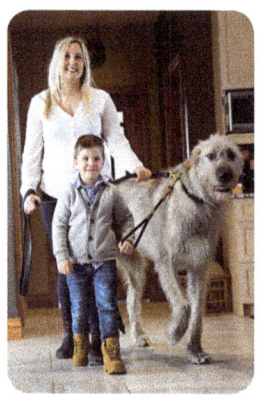

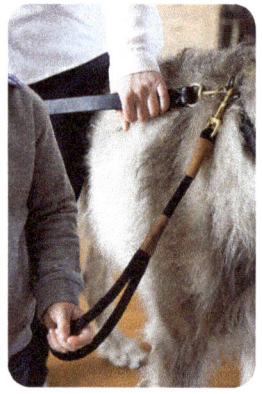

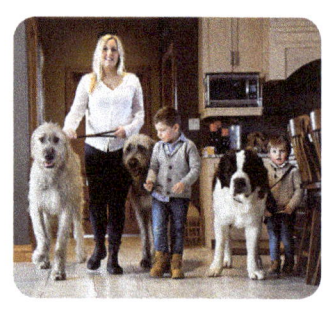

Here, my niece Jody is demonstrating how to properly allow your child to walk a large or giant breed dog. We did this in the house because of the weather conditions but the kids were having fun.

HOW DO I STOP MY DOG FROM JUMPING UP ON ME OR OTHER PEOPLE?

This is something that I find particularly annoying. There is nothing worse than going over to someone's house and getting tackled by their dog! I don't understand why owners tolerate this behavior in their dogs. Would they tolerate that in their children? Would they allow their children to run up and hurl themselves onto their friends in the name of greeting them?

HECK NO they wouldn't! There is absolutely no way on earth that any parent would allow this! So why do they let their dogs get away with it? Why do they brush it off with a nervous "Oh, that's just Fido! He's so happy to see you!"?

It is unacceptable behaviour! PERIOD!

Now, how do you correct it?

If it is a large dog that's jumping up on you, you simply bring your knee up, thus kneeing them in the chest, and in a very deep voice you say *"NO, DOWN!"* and tuck your hands under your armpits and turn your back on the dog, paying him or her no attention.

Lucky's Way

If you have ever watched dogs wrestle, or run at each other, pay attention to how each dog stops the other from jumping on top of them; they get up on their hind legs and bump chests, and the bigger and stronger-chested dog normally wins.

You have to be the bigger, stronger dog in this situation.

But again, you must be consistent. Now, you're not going to haul off and full-force kick the dog, that's not what I'm saying. I'm saying use the force of the dog's momentum to your advantage. You will not hurt the dog. Simply use equal force back and knee him/her in the chest so they get that it's bad.

The reason you tuck your hands away is to show the dog that you are not playing and will not be rewarding him or her with a game or affection. Not until he or she is under control. Dogs see our hands as tools for giving love and affection, as well as to play with (such as playing fetch or tug of war), and therefore when we hide our hands, we are essentially hiding or taking away any implication that we are condoning their behaviour.

HOW DO I STOP MY DOG FROM BARKING AT PEOPLE WHO COME TO MY HOUSE?

It's basic instinct for your dog to protect its territory and family and, really, if your dog is barking, they are doing their job. They are "announcing" that someone is here! Someone is on their territory!

The question should be, How can I get him or her to stop, *on command,* when there's no obvious threat? Now *that's* different.

Scenario one: your BFF is coming over for coffee. She rings the doorbell and your dog barks like crazy. Once you get to the door and recognize it's your friend, you give the command (in a nice deep voice): "That's enough," and at the same time you pull up on your dog's collar and give him or her a jab in the rib cage to switch his or her attention back to you. If your dog is still barking, repeat the process until he or she stops barking and you can put your dog in a sit stay position.

This is when patience is your friend. Waiting for him or her to stop barking and calm down may take a couple of minutes, but this is a training session, so your friend is fine waiting this out, outside the door.

Once your dog is calm, and in a sit stay position, then let your friend enter. As long as your dog hasn't jumped all over your friend, release your dog, and at that point it's up to you if you want to reward with affection and praise or a little treat.

Okay, probably not going to happen that way the first time, so you do it again, immediately. You do it over and over again, for ten minutes a day, for four days in a row, and he or she should pretty much have it down pat. Again, practice makes perfect, so whoever else lives in the house has to do the exact same thing or your training goes out the window.

Remember, your dog is barking because he is in protection mode, so you have to remind him that you do not need protecting, remain calm, deepen your voice, act dominant, and be confident. Give him the stern command, "That's enough. Sit" or put him on a leash and then get control of the situation. Do not praise him! Praise will encourage the aggression! If you start by saying "It's okay, it's okay…" the dog is going to assume you're talking about his aggressive behaviour and it will just become worse.

This is a daily struggle at my house. With four dogs under the age of four, every day is training day. And with four dogs, it's pack mentality, so training tends to go out the window quickly. However, that does not mean I let it go. Barking is not tolerated and neither is aggression.

Now let's say it's a stranger who comes to your door… now what? The same rules can apply, depending on the stranger, of course. I try to keep leashes handy by my door, and I'll clip one on if I feel there may be a threat, just to let the stranger know that my dog may be well-behaved, but he is also very protective. **Never forget that dogs are a very good judge of character and quite often sense things that we don't.**

WHAT DO I DO IF MY DOG GETS SPRAYED BY A SKUNK?

Well, as fate would have it, while I was writing this book Harold got sprayed! Right in the face! Which is the worst! If it's in their eyes, immediately wash them out with water, or eyewash if you have it in your first aid kit. The sooner you can get your dog bathed, the faster you can get the smell off them, and hopefully not spread it all around your house.

The best recipe to use is 500ml (2 cups) of peroxide, 125ml (1/2 cup) baking soda, and 1 tsp dish soap. That's for your average-sized dog. I doubled it for Harold since he's giant-sized, and honestly should have tripled or quadrupled it but didn't have enough peroxide or baking soda on hand for that (rookie mistake). Combine the ingredients together and massage into your dog. Do not pre-soak your dog first. Let this sit for at least five minutes, then rinse off.

And here's my little trick…condition your dog using Moroccan-oil hair mask. In the future when, or if, they get sprayed by a skunk, the oil from the spray seems to just pill off. Plus, your dog will be super soft and smell amazing!

The tricky part is getting the conditioner on your dog's face without getting it in his eyes, so be very careful. Please remember this is a human-grade conditioner, so if your dog has sensitive skin, he or she may react to it. Also, always make sure you get the conditioner rinsed off completely! If not, your dog may start to get super itchy and that's just excruciating for the poor thing. Oh, and I should warn you, the conditioner is quite costly, but the alternative makes it worth it.

There are a couple of other products that you can pick up at your local pet store to help with the smell if it got on your furniture or carpets as well. One is called "Knockout" and it works pretty well. If your dog got sprayed in the mouth, add "Fresh Breath" by Tropiclean to their drinking water and that will help with not only their skunk breath, but with bad breath in general.

BATHING AND GROOMING

While we're on the topic of bathing dogs, let's talk about grooming. All dogs need to be groomed, whether by a professional (as seen in the photos below) or, if you can manage to do it, on your own.

There are breeds with coats that continually grow and therefore need to be cut on a regular basis. These include the poodle (purebred and crossed breeds) and the Bichon Frise and the Portuguese water dog, who both have hair as opposed to fur. It grows like our hair does and needs proper and well-maintained grooming.

Some other breeds that need special grooming practices include the Afghan hound, the Puli, and the Komondor. The Afghan hound is known for its magnificent coat. This breed needs regular bathing and brushing to help keep the coat long and luxurious. The Puli, also known as a Hungarian herding dog, has a corded coat which needs constant attention to keep from becoming matted and dirty. Like the Puli, the Komondor comes from Hungary, but is used as a guard dog for livestock. Their coats are also corded and resemble dreadlocks, which must be kept clean in order for them to appear tidy. This is one breed of dog that is never brushed! Once the cords or dreadlocks are formed, they need to be kept separated in order to prevent matting.

Once again, do as much research as possible on the dog you choose to make sure you are getting one that you can handle.

My boys get bathed and groomed regularly since we go out in public so often and no one likes the smell of dog. If I'm just giving them a quick bath, I use a good quality dog shampoo on them, and then the Moroccan-oil Hair Mask as their conditioner. Over and above that, each time we leave the house to go visiting, I spray them with the new Moroccan-oil body spray. This way, even if we are visiting people who have a sight deficiency, they can still enjoy the smell of my boys along with their super soft coats. Also, they always know it's us, because no one else smells as good as my dogs…or so I've been told many, many times.

If, by chance, you or your dog has a reaction to any grooming products whether it's meant for dogs or humans, stop using it immediately and seek the advice of your Vet. Any dog that is known to have extremely sensitive skin is NOT a dog I would use these products on. In such a case, search out a reputable groomer and ask their advice.

I want to give a quick shout out to my own hair stylist and friend, Gerdina Goodyer, from Mane Attractions in Moncton, Ontario. When she heard that I use these products on my dogs, she allowed me to buy them from her at her cost price, which makes a **huge** difference! She explained to me that it's her way of helping out and doing her part with what my therapy dogs do for others. She knows that I do all of my therapy work free of charge. I'm eternally grateful for her help.

One more point about grooming...Irish Wolfhounds, for example, have wiry outer coats, can be hand-stripped to reveal a soft, smooth undercoat. Hand-stripping is the process of pulling or stripping out of the dead outer coat of the wired hair breeds by hand rather than by cutting the hair with clippers. Hand stripping helps to maintain a proper wire coat, while clipping will ruin the texture of the outer wire coat and the coat colour will change and fade out. Done right, this does not hurt the dogs, in fact, my boys both slept through it. Here are a couple pictures of my groomer hand-stripping Harold and Leonard. It was a lot harder on her than them, that's for sure.

A few things to mention about hand stripping; first, the wire coat is one layer and after stripping that layer off, it's leaving your dog in their thin, soft undercoat until a new wire coat comes through. It may take up to 8 to 10 weeks before the new wire coat fills in again. Next, expect to pay up to double what you would for a regular grooming! This is a labor of love for a most groomers and it can be very hard on the groomer's body. Finally, make sure your dog's coat is ready for hand stripping. It has to be filled in enough, or long enough to get the best finished look.

Finally, here is a list of common breeds that are typically hand stripped:

- Affenpinscher
- Airedale Terrier
- Australian Terrier
- Border Terrier
- Brussels Griffon
- Cairn Terrier
- Dachshund (Wirehaired)
- Irish Terrier
- Irish Wolfhound
- Lakeland Terrier
- Miniature Schnauzer
- Norfolk Terrier
- Otterhound
- Parsons Terrier
- Scottish Deerhound
- Scottish Terrier
- Spinone Italiano
- Standard Schnauzer
- Welsh Terrier
- Wire Fox Terrier
- Wire-haired Pointing Griffon

Brenda Boemer-Groenestege

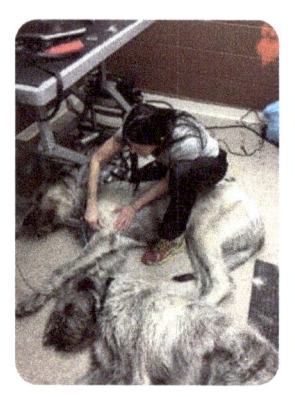

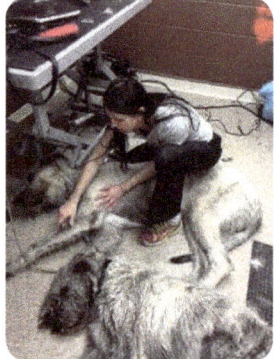

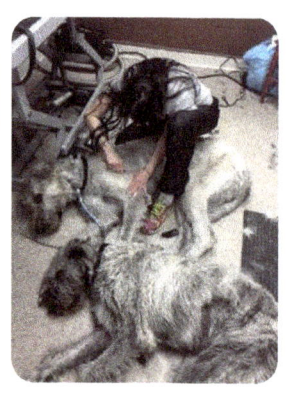

Here is Kirsten Lee, owner of Pin Up Pups Grooming Salon, hand-stripping Harold and Leonard. As you can see, they are sleeping through the entire process.

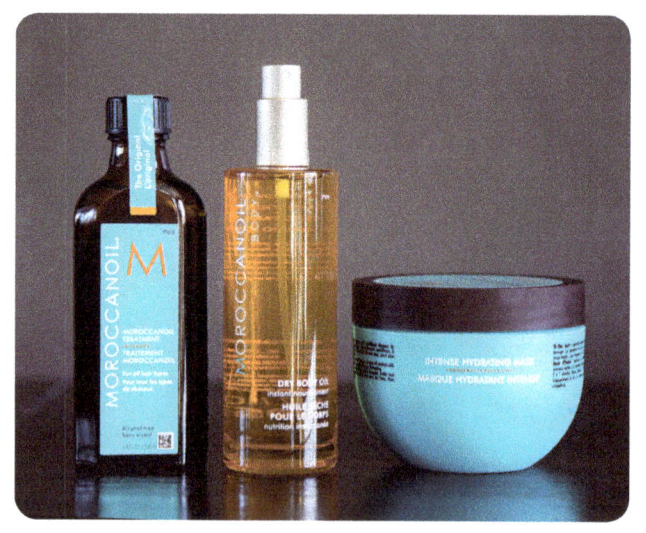

The Moroccan-oil products that make my dogs' fur soft and smell amazing! Thank you, Gerdina!

A TRICK TO HELP ON SLIPPERY FLOORING

My little guy, Clark (when I use the term "little" it's because he's my youngest, not necessarily my smallest), seems to have an issue with our kitchen floor. He whines and cries because he can't get up by himself due to the floor being too slippery…unless, of course, there's food around and then he can pop up, no problem.

Lucky's Way

So, how do you help your giant breed dog get up every time he or she needs to get up? Well, we call it his magic carpet. It's just a 2'x 4' throw rug that I set down in front of Clark whenever he needs to get up. He climbs up on it and boom, he's up.

As he grows, we keep investing in bigger and bigger runners since our floor is so slippery, and he just loves his magic carpets. The newest one I've invested in since writing this book is 2'x 9'.

This would also help geriatric dogs. Although, after a certain point, if your dog is in pain or has arthritis, the magic carpet trick will not work forever.

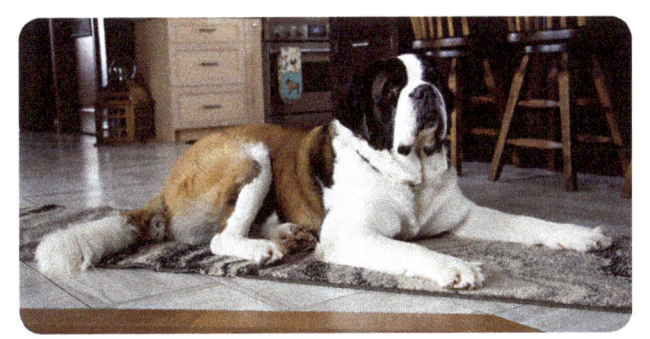

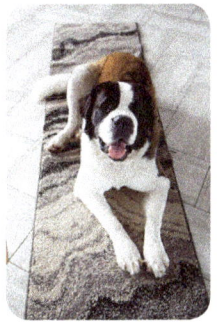

Clark Griswald and his magic carpet.

CHAPTER 9

Lucky's Way...Tips You Won't Find In a Book or on Google

If you are introducing a new baby into the house and you have a dog, and if you are anything like I am and your dog is like a child to you, my father taught me that what you do is bring home the receiving blanket that they wrapped the baby in right after delivery. Yes, you read that correctly, it's the blanket with all the natural scent on it from the first few seconds of your new baby's life. Take that blanket home and give it to your dog.

It really doesn't matter the breed of dog; from an outside guard dog like a Rottweiler or German shepherd to a teacup Yorkshire terrier or Chihuahua, what you're doing is imprinting the smell of your baby into your dog's brain before you even bring that little bundle of joy home. You will be surprised at how protective your dog will be toward your baby.

You should NEVER, ever, chain up a German shepherd! That's the quickest way to turn that breed mean. Put them in a kennel or a dog run of some sort, a fenced-in yard or something, but do not chain them up. Even if it is a mixed-breed shepherd. You will still end up with a mean dog on your hands.

I'll give you the reasoning behind it…putting a German shepherd on a leash puts the dog on automatic guard duty. That's what they're bred for, that's what their natural instincts are, and unless they have proper training and a confident handler on the other end of the leash, they will resort back to those instincts one hundred percent of the time. Put a German shepherd on a chain and what do they think they are doing? Guarding, right! And a guarding shepherd is a very dangerous dog. Put your shepherd into a nice big enclosure and let him or her run free and you have yourself a pet.

Again, do your homework on this breed and for the love of Pete (who the heck is Pete, by the way?), make sure you are getting your German shepherd from a reputable breeder. For this breed of dog, you, as an owner, must have prior experience with dominant breeds and should definitely get help with training if you are not a seasoned dog trainer. They are beautiful, extremely smart, loyal dogs and given the right training will be a wonderful addition to any family. Unfortunately, they can suffer from hip dysplasia and skin disorders like hot spots, but again, searching out the right breeder can be the key to your dog living a long, healthy life.

My dad was the one who taught me the 10–4 method. When teaching your dog to do something new, do it repeatedly for ten minutes every day for four days in a row and it'll have it down pat. The trick is to be very diligent and focused while you're doing the training. Put away your cell phone, ignore your spouse or partner and children, and put all your attention on your dog. Repeat the task that you're teaching him over and over again and always leave a training session on a good note.

If something happens to your puppy before the age of eleven weeks, it will be ingrained in him for life. That's why it's so important to be very careful that your puppy has only good life experiences and positive training practices while he's growing up, because this is when he is most vulnerable and quite often a negative experience haunts both puppy and owners for the life of the dog.

The training of your pup is very important starting at a young age, but it really is all play until the age of seven months. When they reach the seven-month mark, they essentially become a teenager, and then they can retain the more difficult and in-depth training techniques, whether it's for therapy or Schutzhund, or for just being a really well-behaved family pet.

Lucky's Way

If you own a medium, large, or giant breed dog that has even a minuscule amount of aggression in it and it gets a broken leg or needs surgery to fix something, ask your vet beforehand if there's a chance that the dog will have chronic pain issues. Why? A dog in pain has the potential to become a mean dog because of it. They have no way of telling us that they are hurting, so they tend to lash out. If your dog is already showing signs of aggression before the injury, then you are asking for trouble if they will be having chronic pain. You must think of how much pain that dog will be in and what happens, not *if*, but *when*, that dog lashes out. You can only pray that it will be *you* on the receiving end of that bite and not a child, because that would be devastating.

I'm going to introduce you to Bud next. You will understand the relevancy of why I said what I did about your dog lashes out and biting at you at the end of Bud's story.

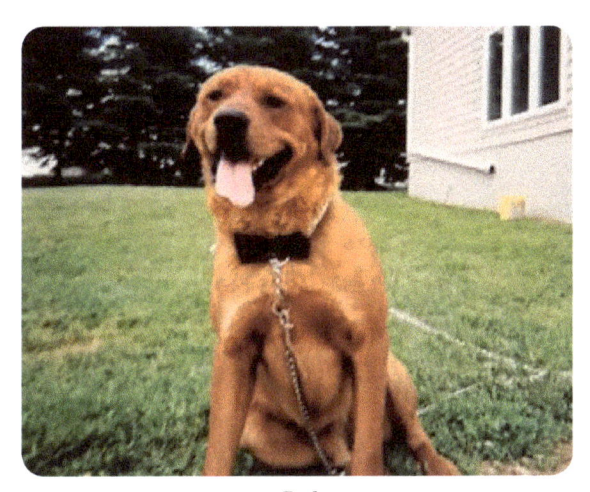

Bud

INTRODUCING BUD
(aka Bob the dog...Robert John when I'm angry,
because all my dogs have two names)
When I first got Bob the puppy, I had to bring him home at five-and-a-half weeks old because the mom Rottweiler was so sick and couldn't feed the puppies and they were just too much for her to handle.

Brenda Boemer-Groenestege

It was Dylan who chose the name Bob. Growing up, Dylan had three goldfish named Bob, Bob, and Bob, and he had a cat named Bob, so when we got this puppy and we talked about names…well, Dylan suggested Bob. I asked him why. What was so special about the name "Bob"? And his response was this: "Mom, think about it, if we're at a park and we can't find our dog and you whistle really loud and then yell, "Here, Bob," chances are a few men might come over but only one dog will come running and that'll be our dog." With a shrug of his shoulders, he smiled at me, happy with his ten-year-old logic, and said "Bob the dog." That's how he got his name.

I brought my new puppy over on a Sunday morning in January: January 12, 2002, to be exact. To meet my dad. My Uncle Bernie was there for coffee, which was pretty normal (you remember Bernie, right? He drove me to the airport to pick up the German shepherd who kicked my ex's ass?). Anyhow, my dad said to Bernie, "That's the best dog she's ever going to own." Little did I know that those were going to be the very last words I would ever hear my father say. I would never hear his voice again.

I went home giddy from hearing him say such an amazing thing. The next morning I got the call at work. The call that changed my life forever. My dad had had a massive stroke. He had an aneurysm burst in the base of his brain stem. He lay in a coma for three days before he died. I never left his side in the hospital for more than half an hour to go home and shower. He was sixty-seven years old. My whole world changed. I still miss him every day.

Later that spring, when I first started dating my now-husband, Bob, the funniest thing was telling him I had a dog named Bob. After most dates, my boyfriend, Bob, would drop me off and say to me, "Will you please change your dog's name?" and I'd say, "Nope, not until you prove to be as faithful as he is."

We thought this was really funny but my boyfriend Bob…well, not so much. Anyway, after boyfriend Bob asked us to move in (when I say "us," I mean my kids [Spencer and Dylan], a black Lab named Bailey, Bob the dog, and myself), one of the first things he asked me was, "Now will you change the damn dog's name?" I laughed and said, "Yes, but it's going to be difficult because it's habit now that when I'm pissed off at him I yell '*Robert John*, get over here!' But the boys and I did talk about it already and we agreed that we can call him Budweiser or Bud for short. Happy?"

Well! The look on boyfriend Bob's face was a combination of shock and confusion. He was looking at me with his beer halfway to his open mouth when I asked him, somewhat frustrated, "What? You don't like the name Bud either?"

He started shaking his head. "What did you say you call him when you're pissed off?" "Robert John," I replied. Then I started attempting to explain to a non-dog person why all my dogs have a middle name. He sat there staring at me like I was crazy so I finally just sat back and huffed "WHAT?"

Bob said to me, "Holy crap, it's going to get confusing around here, that's for sure!" He finished with, "Do you have any idea what my full name is?"

Okay, now you know what's coming, right? Oh yeah…I started laughing, like pee-your-pants laughing! Sulking, Bob starts in with, "It's not that funny! How would you like to have the same name as a dog? You can stop laughing anytime now!"

I caught my breath and finally stopped laughing. I said, "Hey, listen honey, at least you have a nice first and middle name. Wait until I tell you what mine is. You may rethink this whole moving-in-together business altogether. It's that bad!"

Bob was looking at me very skeptically. "I don't believe you at all! Now you're going to make up some stupid name just to make me feel better!"

"Umm, yeah, NO, I don't have to do that; my middle name is THAT bad! Ready? Wait for it…Henrietta! Isn't that a beauty? My sisters had a chicken and called her Henrietta and my whole childhood they told me I was named after a chicken, so yes, I do understand, Bob." I had to get my driver's license out to prove it to him.

Anyhow, back to our dog. Over the years, Bud was a 130-pound killing machine! There wasn't a raccoon, rabbit, stray cat, muskrat, etc. that Bud wouldn't take on.

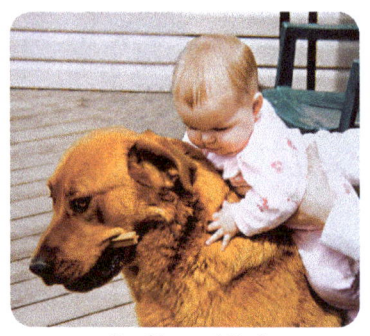

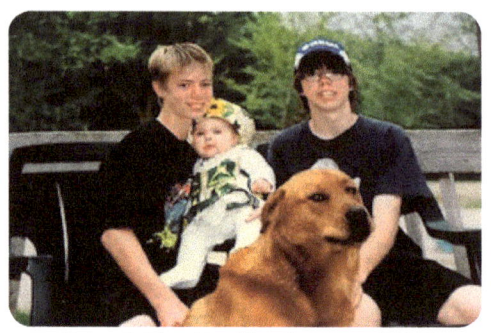

Brooklyn and Bud   *Dylan, holding Brooklyn, Spencer, and Bud*

    Bud also sat patiently as Brooklyn applied makeup on him when she was younger. He would sit as still as can be while she smeared lipstick all over his mouth and mascara and eye shadow on his eyes, and then she would dress him up and he'd sit on a chair behind her and play bus driver for as long as she wanted him to. He was extremely patient with her and very protective of her as well.

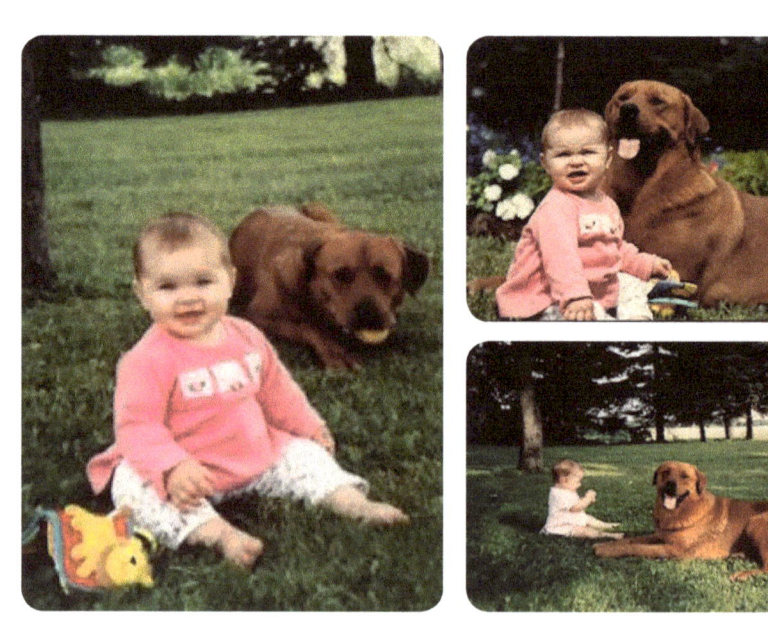

It was hard finding baby pictures without Bud in them.

It was Thanksgiving. Brooklyn was just under two years old that year and we were having Bob's family over for dinner. I've never been more thankful for a big family than I was that year!

We had just built a small barn for our two horses. Bob's brother Henry and his wife Johanne live just down and across the road from us about half a mile or so, on a pig farm, and they had just bought a cow and calf and everyone was going down to see them, including Bob and Brooklyn. Then they were all coming back to our house to see our horses and eat dinner.

We expected forty to forty-five people at our house for dinner, so to say I was a little *distracted* in the kitchen would be an understatement.

Anyhow, Bob came in and I asked him where Brooklyn was and he said, very nonchalantly, "She came in the house."

"No, she didn't," I said, and others around me helping in the kitchen agreed. He was adamant he saw her heading for the house, so he figured she came in.

That's when I was super thankful for a big family because once word got out that Brooklyn was missing *ALL HELL BROKE LOOSE!*

The scariest thing about country living is when there is a mature corn field and a missing toddler! We were all screaming her name, but nothing! She was nowhere!

Finally, I realized something; Bud was missing too! I told everyone to stop shouting for a minute and I whistled as loud as I could. We heard Bud bark!

I've never seen my husband run so fast EVER!

There they were: our little girl, ACROSS the road, in the ditch, walking, halfway between us and Uncle Henry's house, with Bud faithfully walking between her and the road.

When Bob caught up to her he asked her where she was going and she simply replied "to see Uncle Henry cow." That Thanksgiving we gave thanks, all right, and Bud got the biggest ham bone *ever*!

Unfortunately, we lost Bailey, my black Lab, about a year after moving in with Bob, when she ingested rat poison that had been left in one of the old barns. We didn't know it was there until it was too late.

When Brooklyn was three years old, we put an in-ground pool in. The contractor who installed it pointed out to us that whenever Brooklyn walked by the pool, Bud would automatically walk between her and the water. Neat, eh?

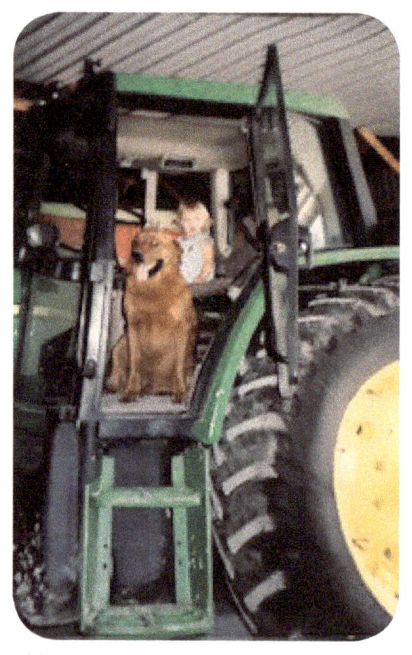

Brooklyn and Bud...he was always with her, always!

Bud had an active life; he would frequently go off, chasing deer and other things, and he quite often came home with one injury after another that needed tending too. I had made my dad a promise: if I owned a big dog and if that dog had a serious injury, like a broken bone or something equally bad, then we euthanize him. Thankfully, I haven't had to make that choice… yet. Bud made the choice for me one day. He chose his own fate, unfortunately.

One time we watched Bud drag home a deer carcass. Yep, a whole carcass! Local hunters had stripped it and then left it behind and Bud decided to bring it home to chew on. It sure kept the door to door soliciting down for a while. Nothing like having a huge dog chomping on a bloody carcass right beside your driveway to dissuade unwanted guests from popping in.

We did notice that occasionally Bud would limp and we figured he got hurt either on the chase or maybe on the road.

Lucky's Way

When we first moved in with Bob, "*Dogs belong outside on the farm!*" That was non-negotiable. To be quite honest, after being a single mom for ten years, I was okay with it. Life for me had been hard, and moving in with Bob was like a dream come true. So coming to terms with having to keep my dogs outside, where they actually wanted to be, was not hard.

Bob is an amazing and talented carpenter and he built my dogs beautiful heated dog houses, so they were just fine outside. And the more comfortable I got living here, well, let's just say the dogs slowly made their way into the house, on occasion, and there were a lot of occasions.

I have to give credit where credit is due. My mother, Margret Boemer, taught me so many things. My love of cooking, my talent for entertaining, and always being the best mom you can be to your kids! But my favourite thing my mom said to me has to be this, "You know, Brenda, it doesn't matter how big or strong your husband is, or even how smart he *thinks* he is, you just have to let him know he *is* the head of the family…but *you, you are the neck!*"* *Thanks Mom!*

*The neck turns the head wherever it wants it to go, thus controlling it.

Case in point, when Bud was around six, I started noticing that he was slowing down, which is normal for large or giant breed dogs. What they call "quality of life" starts to falter for the giant breeds anywhere after four to six years of age, depending on the breed. Check with your breeder before buying one of the really, really heavy breeds like the Old English Mastiff or the heavy-coated Saint Bernard.

At the time, Bob was working at a neighbouring farmer's house and they had a Saint Bernard. Every day he would come home and tell me how amazing this dog was. Apparently, as a young boy, he would beg his parents to get him one. I was never a big fan of them. They're hairy, with lots of drool, they're known to be stubborn, and quite frankly, it just wasn't the breed I had on my personal bucket list of dogs.

I started talking to Bob about possibly getting another dog because Bud was slowing down. My theory on this is that, at his age, he was still young enough to teach the puppy good habits, but old enough not to teach him the bad stuff, like taking off on hunting excursions for hours on end—or so I thought.

As anticipated, Bob's immediate answer was emphatically, "*NO WAY! We do NOT need another dog!*"

To my dog lover's ears, it sounded distinctly like, "Maybe…possibly, I'll consider it…that sounds like a good idea." You just have to read between the lines a bit.

The very next day I was in the office paying bills, and for some strange reason, in our personal handwritten phonebook (for you young people, that's a small journal-like book with alphabetized pages, on which you write down the names and phone numbers of friends, family, business associates, etc.), and what did I find? The name and phone number of a Saint Bernard breeder! Crazy, right? Coincidence? I think not! It was Fate, I tell you! I remembered then that I had seen an ad in the newspaper a few years earlier when a friend of mine wanted to get a Saint Bernard for her daughter, so I had jotted down the number.

I stared at that phone number for a good thirteen seconds! I'm serious! It could have even been closer to fourteen seconds! I put a lot of thought into it before I picked up the phone and called the number.

It rang and rang. Finally a gentleman picked up. I excitedly said, "Hello, sir…I found your number in my Rolodex file. I had jotted it down from an ad in the paper. It's going back a few years, but it's about some Saint Bernard puppies. You wouldn't possibly have any puppies now, by chance, would you?"

I swear my heart stopped beating while I waited for him to answer my question. Could fate actually have put this man's phone number in my hands at the exact time that he had puppies? After all these years? I took one desperately needed breath and then he gave me my soul-crushing answer, "Uh, no, I don't got any puppies no more. I haven't bred my bitch in quite some time," he explained in his methodical Mennonite drawl.

What! Did I hear that correctly? My head was spinning! I was so certain that it was meant to be! I was meant to find his number! Fate wanted me to call him! He was supposed to have puppies and wham, just like that, I'd have a new puppy by suppertime! What the heck happened? My puppy fantasy from three minutes earlier had just died.

I honestly didn't know what to say to him after that. I was stunned. Shocked. I felt light-headed. There was dead air on the phone.

"Ah, you still there, lady?" he asked.

"Oh, yes, I'm sorry," I began to reply. He interrupted me and began talking again in his methodical Mennonite drawl, "Now, I sold a bitch from my last litter to my milk (he pronounces it "melk") truck driver and she did have a litter of eleven really healthy pups and I'm pretty sure they're ready to go. Why, I talked to him just the other day when he was here pickin' up 'melk' and I'm thinkin' there were still some available. If yer wanten I can probably go find his number for ya?"

I jumped out of my chair. "YES, PLEASE! I would love his number, thank you!" I tried not to yell through the phone to *hurry the heck up and get the darn number*, because patience isn't really one of my strong suits, and waiting for him was getting increasingly difficult as the seconds ticked by.

Eventually, he did return and rhymed off the ten-digit number at an excruciatingly slow pace.

I made the call to the milk truck driver's wife and found out that, yes, she did indeed have puppies, and **yes! yes! yes!** there were indeed still some available pups.

Again, patience not being my strong suit, this resulted in me not actually waiting and thinking it through thoroughly, but rather jumping in my truck and calling ahead to Brooklyn's school and telling the secretary (my good friend Judi) what was going on. Then I was on my way to pick Brooklyn up so we could go and "look" at the puppies.

"Yeah, right," Judi said, laughing at me. She knew darn well we were coming home with one.

Off Brooklyn and I went. We had already picked out his name, so we just had to find the matching puppy. Names seem to come to me before I ever get a puppy. Quite often actually, it's the name that prompts the getting of the new puppy. That's my sign. When I suddenly hear a name that resonates with me as an awesome dog name… well, that's when I start the search for the matching dog begins.

If you are ever down in the dumps and you need a mood booster, do yourself a favour and find a litter of Saint Bernard puppies! It's cuteness overload.

Brenda Boemer-Groenestege

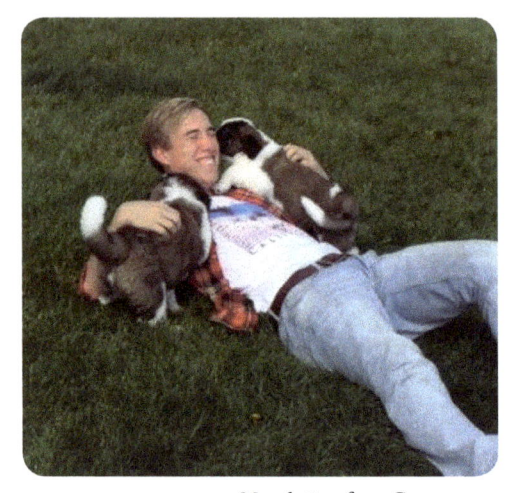

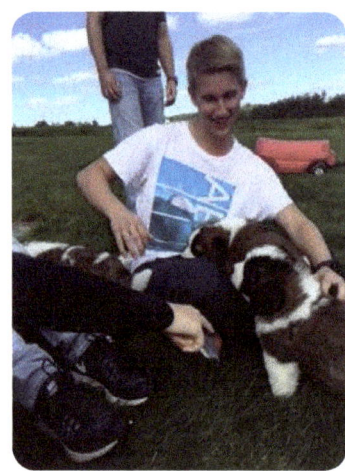

My relatives from Germany were in heaven when we went to visit Clark Griswald and his siblings.

When we got there, in the yard stood the most beautiful Swiss chalet dog kennel. It was amazing. A scene right out of the movie *George* (again, millennials, just google it). It was the size of a large two-story tool shed, painted in the red and white colours of Switzerland, and included fake snow on the alps. Stunning.

There, in the yard, were so many cute Saint Bernard puppies to choose from it was difficult to not take them all home! Finally, I had picked my puppy, but a different puppy had apparently picked Brooklyn! She was right, of course, when she said, "Mom, *this* is our puppy! *This is TRUMAN!*" And, gosh darnit, he was all kinds of awesome!

As we drove home, the realization began to set in that within minutes I was going to have to confront Bob with a new puppy that he had explicitly said he "absolutely *did not want!*" What was I going to do? Seriously, how angry would he be? I mean, now Brooklyn has fallen head over heels in love with Truman and if Bob loses his "you know what," well, Truman may have to go back to the breeder and Brooklyn will be heartbroken. Oh Lord, I really should have thought things through!

The closer we got to home, the more my anxiety built. Brooklyn was also starting to express doubt about bringing our new puppy home. She said, "Dad's going to be really mad, isn't he, Mom?" and asked, "Is he going to make us take Truman back?"

I tried to reassure her, telling her that we'd just slowly tell Dad. Maybe she could just hide him in her room until I poured Dad two or three really stiff whiskies to make sure he was in a better mood before surprising him? What a shining example of motherhood I was, eh?

Brooklyn looked skeptical, to say the least. When we pulled up to our house, as luck would have it Bob was standing right there in the driveway, watching as we drove in. Damn. I had to face the music. I mean, it's only a puppy, right? It's not like it's a horse. Believe it or not, I've done that too and he didn't divorce me.

Well, here goes nothing, I thought. I got out, walked over to him, and put Truman in Bob's arms like you would cradle a baby. I said, with hopeful eyes, as sweet as can be, "Meet our new puppy. His name is Truman."

Bob looked at me, then looked down at Truman and back to me again. His face lit up and he said, "I can't believe you bought a Saint Bernard!" That was it! It was love at first sight.

Bob physically carried Truman around like a baby until he got too big to carry any longer. It was hilarious and a little bit ridiculous at the same time.

Oh, and the rule of no dogs allowed in the house went right out the window.

Spencer, Dylan, and I would stand in the kitchen and watch our 6'4" tough-as-they-come farmer turn into a baby-talking, cooing, puddle of a puppy lover, holding Truman on his lap and treating him as though he was a newborn gift from above. We would shake our heads and the kids would say, "Maybe he has a brain tumour, Mom, and that's why he's acting like this?" For some men, it's their children that brings out the best in them, but for our man/husband/father, it was finally getting the dog he had wanted since he was a child.

Now, he did stress that he wasn't impressed that I didn't discuss it with him beforehand and that in the future I should always talk to him about getting a dog *before* actually bringing it home with me. At the time I agreed, but truth be known, I've surprised Bob quite often since then with more puppies and the last one almost caused a divorce…almost. I'll tell that story in a bit… it involves Clark Griswald.

Truman was Bob's buddy! Especially when he'd been drinking. That's when it always got funny. Bob would be down on the floor wrestling around with Truman, and Truman just loved it. Nights that Bob had had a few extra whiskies because of a particularly bad week meant extra love for Truman. Bob would crouch down, hanging out our back door, teetering on the edge, and sing (between drunken hiccups), "How much is that doggie in the window?"

There were the nights we would go out to dances, weddings, dinner, wherever, and Bob would have a few drinks (okay, he was drunk), and he'd lovingly say to me, "Honey, I just love that no matter where we go—hiccup—I always have the prettiest girl in the room."

I would think to myself, "Aww, isn't that sweet?" Biased, yes, he's my husband, but nonetheless lovely to hear.

Then, one night, after having a particularly good time at our friend's wedding reception, Bob came home and had a drunken wrestling match on the floor with Truman. Afterward, Bob crawled into bed and wrapped his arms around me ever so gently. He reeked exceptionally strongly of whiskey and onions, compliments of an open bar and the midnight snack he had helped himself to (which included a make-your-own kaiser bar).

After Bob was nicely snuggled into me, he started chatting up a storm about the wedding, and our friends, and finally he got to the speech that I selfishly loved hearing. I know that sounds awful, but my husband isn't one to throw around words of love very easily, and therefore I'll take it when and wherever I can get it.

There we were, in bed, snuggled up, and I'm lying there smiling in the dark because I know what's coming. He's breathing, right in my face, "Honey, I just can't—hiccup—seriously, honey, I just can't—hiccup—oh, s'cuse me, damn hiccups, honey, I just can't believe—hiccup—Honey, I just can't believe how much I love that f**king dog!"

And just like that, I was no longer the prettiest girl in the room.

Lucky's Way

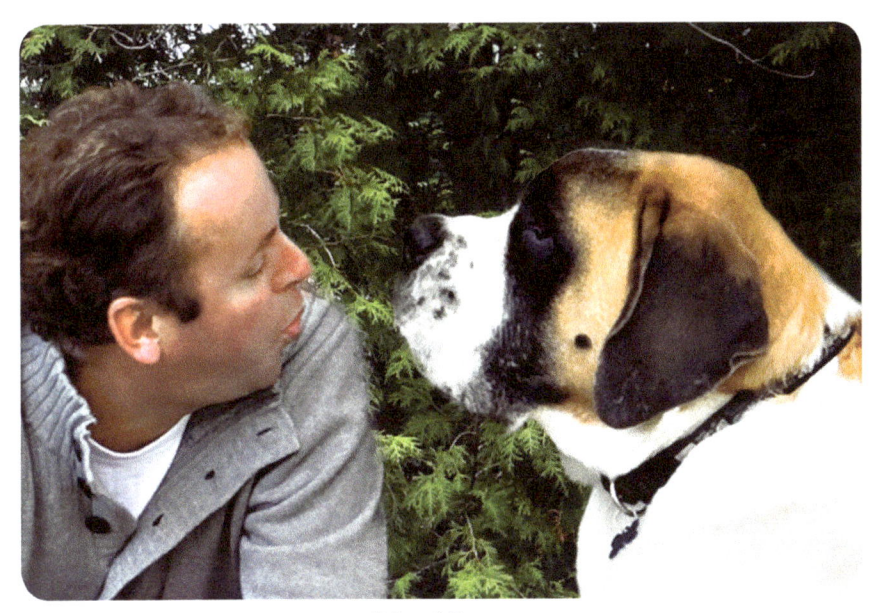

Bob and Truman

On the topic of getting people pets as gifts…it's not the best idea unless you are one hundred percent sure that it's the right decision to make. I've gotten really, really lucky with my husband when it comes to surprising him with a new puppy. But it almost resulted in divorce on more than one occasion in our household, so I DO NOT recommend anyone buying a pet as a gift for someone else.

Brenda Boemer-Groenestege

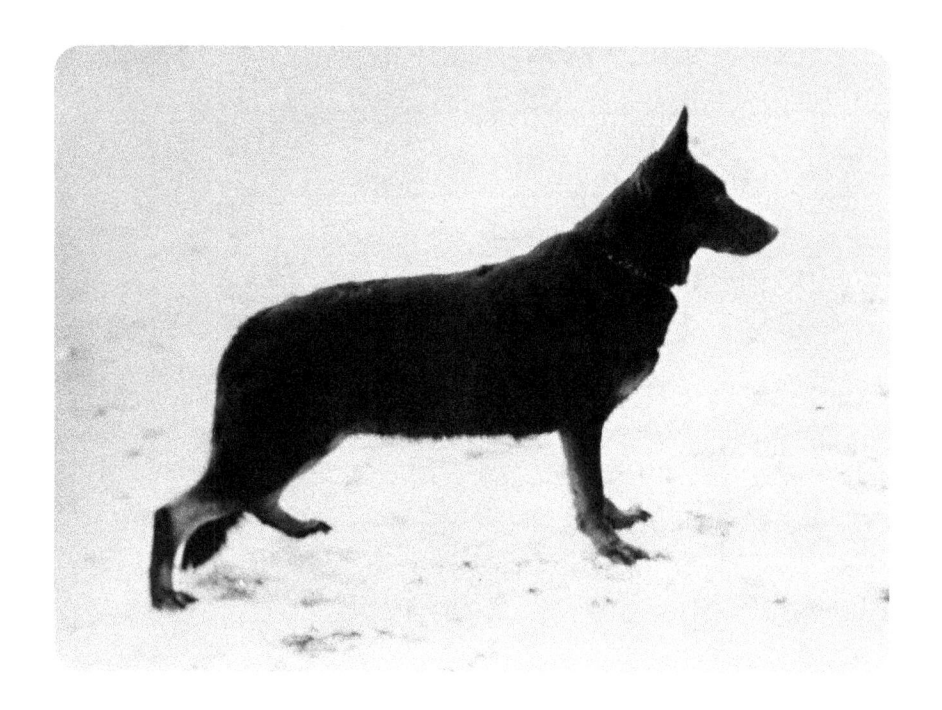

Asta, the legend!
Stories About Lucky and His Dog, Asta

In doing research for my book, I took a trip to Germany to visit my relatives and sat down with my uncles to get a sense of who my father was as a young man. My dad's brothers Franz and Alfons love to tell story after story about my father and the crazy things him and his friends would do. I was left with the distinct impression that my dad, for all intensive purposes, was quite the troublemaker in his own right. Something he never shared with us, his own children. He always came across as such a strict 'wake up at dawn and work until you drop' kinda man. But now, to hear that he was actually my grandparents problem child! Well, now that makes so much sense why he and I were always so close! We were kindred spirits!

My uncle Alfons tells the story of my dad and his friend taking off one weekend on their bicycles (because back then only the rich had motorized vehicles). They would ride throughout the countryside until dark, then find a farmer and ask if they could stay on their farm and in exchange for room and board for the night, they would help by working on the farm. This went on for a couple months! "A couple months!!" I repeated to my uncle, "what did Oma and Opa say when dad finally came home? Were they not worried sick about him?"

"Yes, naturally they were worried about him, but Lucky didn't care. He didn't care about anything or anyone back then. Not until he got introduced to the German shepherds. Then he finally found something he cared about!" My uncle replied.

He watched and learned quickly. Soon it became very apparent that he had a knack with dogs. He started with a dog named Bessie. She was a beautiful, smart, predictable dog. Then, he met Asta. She was almost untrainable. Small, sleek, cunningly smart and deadly, if he wasn't careful. My father fell in love for the first time in his life.

The bond that my dad and Asta would form moving forward together, would be one for the history books. But I credit Asta for turning my father into a man. Would he still drive my grandparents crazy? Absolutely! But she grounded my dad. Asta gave him a purpose when he had no idea what life expected of him. Remember, this was the early 1950's in Germany. They were still very much recovering from the second world war so a lot of people were feeling much the same way as my father. There was still a sense of unease in the air for a lot of people. When my dad found something that he could focus on and ultimately thrive at doing, my grandparents were thrilled. When word got out that my dad had a way of working with and training the "hard to handle", "difficult", or "impossible" dogs, well, that's when he started working hand in hand with the German Police Department.

When my parents began dating, my mom said that Asta came with them on all of their dates. She recounts the story of going for walks with dad and Asta in Greven, the town in Germany where we come from. She said people would always give them a very wide girth because they all knew the stories about Asta, and how, not only was she protective and smart, but also how incredibly dangerous she could be if you challenged her or my father.

The story Mom loves sharing with us, is when dad would put Asta in a sit stay position at the base of church steps, in the centre of town. Dad unclipped her leash and he and mom would leave. They continued walking, and walking, and walking. Mom said it drove her wild that they walked so far and she would beg him to call her!"I think you should call her now Lucky! It's been so far! You must call her! Please Lucky!" She said she would plead with him and he would just get that grin on his face, and keep walking. Mom said finally, FINALLY, after what seemed liked an eternity he would let out one swift, loud whistle and just like that, you could see her running through the town! "It was like watching a black bullet," mom said "ZOOM!! just like that!! And she'd be right beside him again like nothing happened. He'd snap on the leash and away we'd walk." My mom's face glows when she tells that story.

Here are a couple more stories about the incomparable Asta!

WHAT THEY STARTED…SHE WOULD FINISH!

My dad and his friends were out in a pub in Germany, and a group of men came in and started harassing some of the patrons. Of course, my dad chose to get involved and told the men that they were no longer welcome in the pub, and that if they didn't leave, they would be helped out.

When my father and his friend came out of the pub a few hours and a lot of pints of beer later, the same men my father had told to leave were waiting for him outside. Their main target was my dad because he was the guy that kicked them out and now, apparently, they were going to get some payback.

They started taking turns beating him up. They held his friend back, so he couldn't help him. His friend finally fought enough to get free and ran off.

The men were saying, "Oh, what a good friend you have, he just took off and left you here to take a beating! Now we're going to slowly beat you until you beg us to stop!" and then they laughed and laughed. (This is when my dad would get a twinkle in his eye when he was telling the story.)

Dad said he started to laugh too, and they stopped, looked at each other, and then said to him, "What the hell are you laughing at? Is your brain so beat up that you're crazy now?"

Lucky's Way

My dad just said, "Wait for it, she's coming, and then I'll be laughing and you'll be begging me to stop her." The men looked at each other and had no idea what my dad was talking about.

His friend ran to my father's house. When he got there, Dad's German shepherd, Asta, was already going crazy because she sensed that he was in trouble. As soon as he opened her kennel door, she tore out to go help my dad. He was her world, and she knew he was in trouble. Witnesses said that it was like watching lightning strike! That was how fast she ran.

When she got there, she threw herself onto the first man, who had his fist in mid-air to punch my dad again. Dad said he heard the crunch of bones and the man screamed in pain. She then turned to the next one and grabbed him by his shoulder because he was holding my dad. Another scream ripped through the air. The third man tried to kick Asta when she came toward him, and that ended up with him writhing in pain since, as witnesses told my dad later, she was so smart that when he missed her, she simply grabbed him right in the back of the thigh and shook him until he too was screaming.

The last of the group decided to try to run away, but that was not going to happen either. You see, if you have my father's blood on your hands, let's just say you're in the line of fire because his dog is out for payback! And you cannot outrun a German shepherd! She ran after him, caught him by the back of his ankle, and again, from witnesses relaying the story, you could hear the bones crunch from quite a distance away.

My father said he could barely see at this point because his eyes were so swollen but he could hear the men screaming in pain and begging for him to call her off. He did. Her work was done. Between his friend and Asta, he managed to get home. But then he had to face my Oma (his mom). He said, with a grin, "That was worse than the beating!"

HE THOUGHT SHE WAS DEAD!

Taking your dog into the pub with you in Germany is very common even now, and years ago, on this particular day, my dad had brought Asta in with him. It started out like any other Saturday, my father said; he and Asta were in the local pub enjoying a beer with some of his friends. Asta was lying faithfully and quietly beside him as she usually did. Then, a stranger walked in and sat at my dad's table, right beside where Asta was lying down.

Now, the town where my parents come from in Germany isn't very big. So everyone pretty much knows each other. This gentleman who had just sat down at the table was a complete stranger to my dad.

"Huh, so this is the famous dog, eh?" he said.

"What are you talking about?" my dad asked him.

"This dog? Asta, right? This is the famous Asta?" the man said, quite sarcastically.

Now the entire pub was watching to see what was going on. My dad couldn't figure out what this man wanted.

Dad said, "This is Asta, yes. I don't know why you're calling her famous. But this is my dog, yes, so what? What do you want?"

At this point the man stood up and started to get a bit dramatic, waving his arms around while he talked. "Oh, she's famous all right! Hasn't she won all the awards? Hasn't she beaten so many other dogs in the ring to be the number one dog? Isn't she supposed to be the smartest dog around?"

Dad said he just sat there and watched the guy. No one really knew what to do or say, so they just watched.

"Well, huh, she doesn't look that smart to me! In fact, she looks kind of stupid! And she sure doesn't look very tough! I don't know what all the talk is about! She just looks like a dumb, stupid dog!"

And with that, he picked up a chair and smashed it over Asta's head! Completely knocking her out cold! My dad was in absolute shock. He told me he *thought the man had killed her*!

I asked my father if he beat the living hell out of the man. He said no, he was so worried about his dog that he didn't even care about the man at that point. He just concentrated on Asta.

As he recounted the story to me, I could see the anger in my dad's eyes. Dad looked right at me and said, "I sought she vas dead! She just lay dere not moving! I sought that son of a bitch killed her!" The pain was still there after all these years. He shook his head and continued.

The man was laughing his head off when he left the pub.

It took weeks before Asta recovered completely from that trauma. Back then, they didn't do x-rays or anything like that on their dogs, so it was just strictly keeping an eye on her and hoping and praying that she would get better.

Life went on, and dad said he would occasionally think about the man, but he never saw him again until almost a year later, when, just like that, the same guy walked into the same pub and sat down in the same chair. Asta was sleeping beside my dad on the floor, just like before, and this man came in and sat down right beside her!

Dad said he was just about to say, "You've got a lot of nerve coming in here" when all of a sudden, the man screamed in pain. Dad looked down at Asta and she was still fast asleep, so he turned to the man and said, "What's wrong with you?"

"Your dog just bit me!" he screamed.

Once again, dad looked down at Asta, who was still lying calmly beside him, but now she was looking at my dad. Dad said he gave Asta a little nod and she quickly put her head down and closed her eyes again.

Then he said to the stranger, "I don't think so. Look at her, she's sleeping."

The man pulled his sleeve up and there was a huge piece of muscle hanging off his arm. Dad said it was really gross.

"You should get that looked at by a doctor," Dad said calmly.

"Your dog did this! I want that dog killed! It's a monster! Everyone in here saw it bite me, right?!" the man screamed.

Funny thing about small towns, no one seemed to see anything. "We saw you try to kill the dog when you hit her over the head with a chair," the pub owner said, and everyone agreed.

The stranger left that day and was never seen in their little town again.

ASTA ALWAYS FINDS THE THIEF!

On more than one occasion, the police came calling on my father in the middle of the night, needing his help. Of course, it was his dog's help that they were after. She was an exceptional search dog.

Asta could search out anything and anyone. My favorite story, which my uncle told me, was when the police called on my dad and Asta one night to come out and search for a thief.

When my dad got there, the owner of the property was very upset, blaming the theft on his neighbours, who were jealous of him and his family. The owner was parading around like a peacock, thinking and acting like he was so much classier than anyone else and showing off how important he was, living in a big house with his wife and son. Everyone wanted to have what he had, and he could trust no one!

Apparently, it was quite the show. So my dad and Asta started where the theft began, which was in the house, of course, and right away Asta caught a scent.

She was running with the scent, my uncle told me, his eyes lit up, and she and my dad ran, with the police in tow, around the back, into the shed, then out of the shed, then back around to the front of the house again, and once more around to the back behind the shed, before coming in through the back door.

"What is that dog doing?!" the strutting peacock man demanded.

"She's following the scent of the thief," the police chief told him.

"There's something wrong with that dog. It must have lost the scent. Why did it go back into the house? Obviously it's not a very good dog. Go get a better dog!" he demanded.

The police chief told him, "She is the number one dog in all of Germany for tracking. She will find the thief. I guarantee it!"

Once again, Asta came outside and followed the scent. But she seemed confused. My dad called the police chief over and quietly explained what he thought had happened. Just as he was doing this, a car with a group of young men pulled up. It was the son of the owner of the property and his friends, home from a night at the pub.

Suddenly, Asta went crazy! She tried to grab the son's leg. The son ran into the house. Dad and Asta went after him.

Peacock man was screaming, "What are you doing? That is my son!"

The police chief said, "I told you she would find the thief, didn't I? Your son is the thief, sir!"

"WHAT! NO! You're lying! It can't be! It's not possible," he said.

When they all came back out of the house, the police had the son in custody, and they had found most of the stolen items hidden in the son's room.

Lucky's Way

Suddenly the man wasn't feeling so boastful anymore.

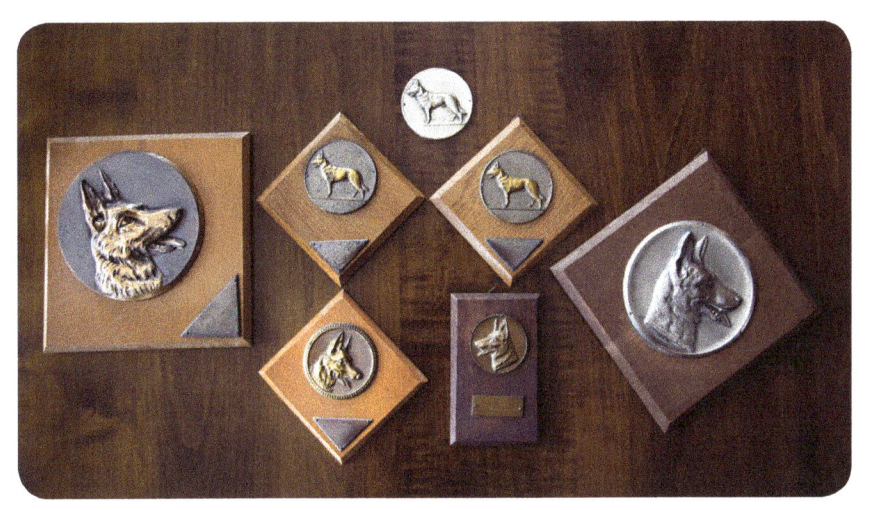

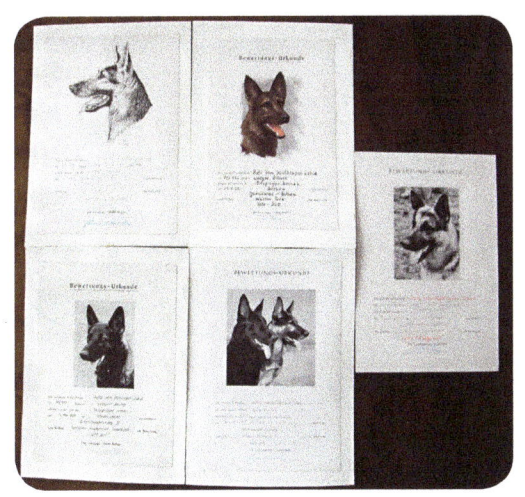

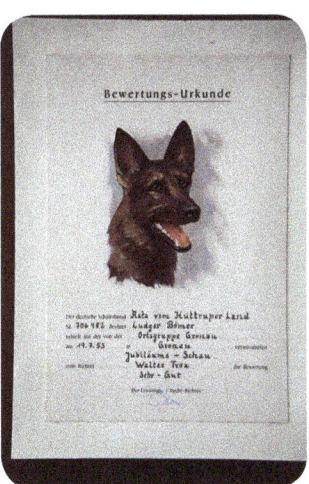

*These were found in my Oma's attic when I went to
Germany to gather stories for my book*

CHAPTER 10

Stories and Pictures from GG Therapy Dogs

Young or Young at Heart, Love is Love When it Comes to Dogs

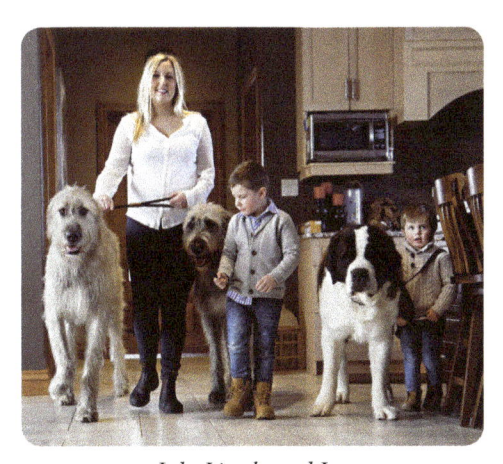

Jody, Lincoln, and Leo

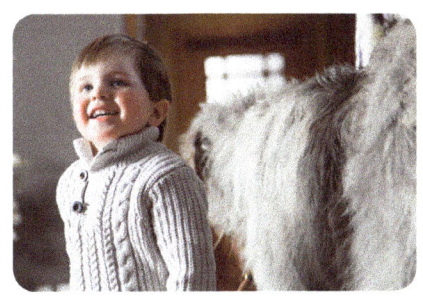

Leo with Harold

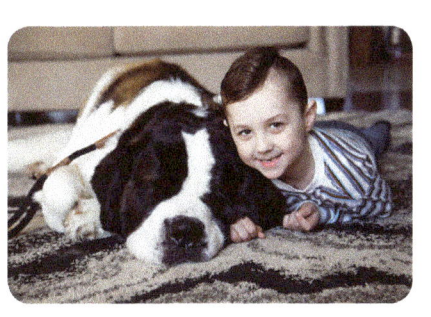

Ryder and Clark Griswald

163

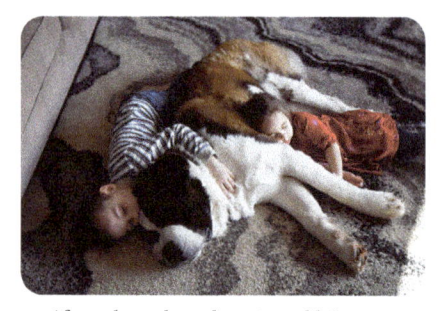

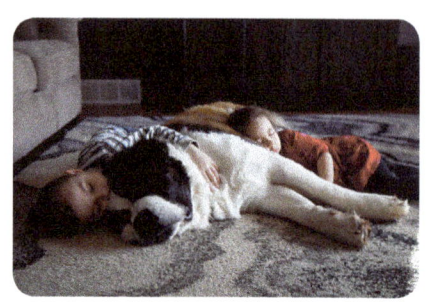

After a long photo shoot, it couldn't get any cuter than this...Ryder, Ayla, and Clark Griswald.

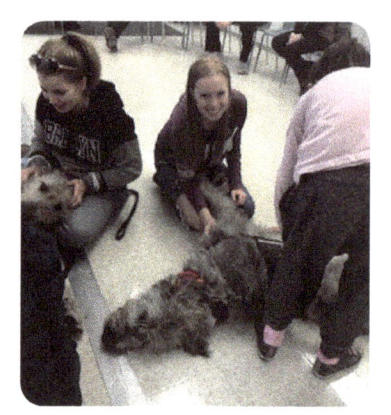

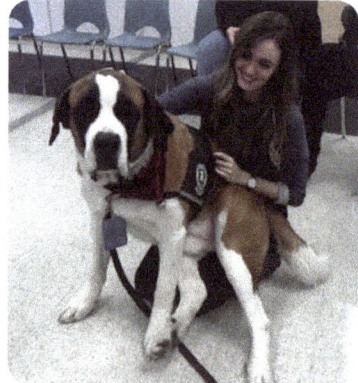

The students at Mitchell District High School love when we visit.

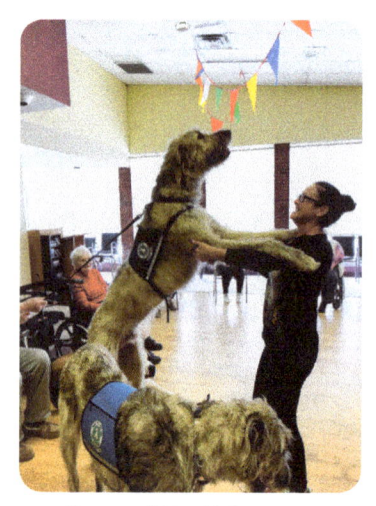

Karen and Harold dancing at group therapy

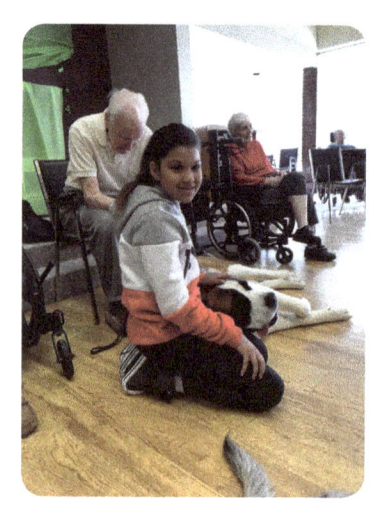

Myah certainly enjoys when Lloyd visits her mom's work

Lucky's Way

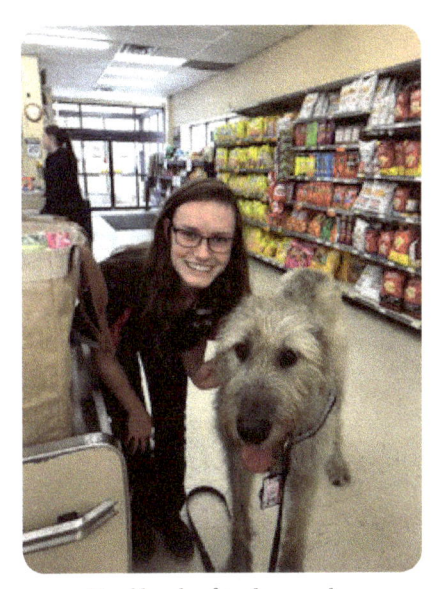

*Harold makes friends everywhere,
even the grocery store*

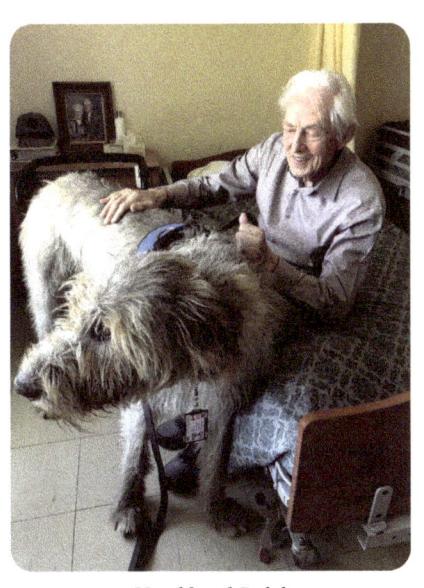

Harold and Ralph

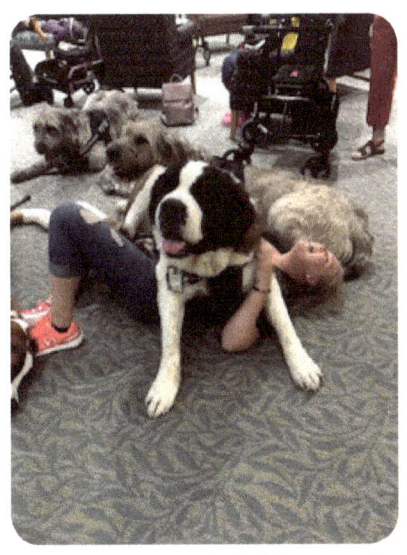

Alisha is in heaven with Clark laying over her

Brenda Boemer-Groenestege

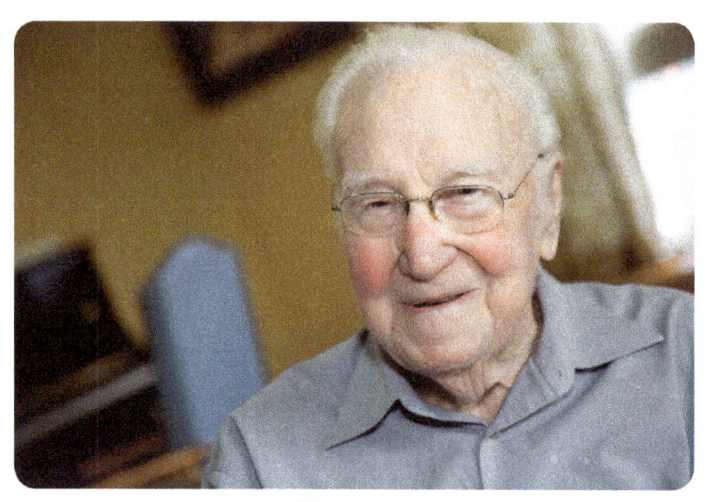

Walter's Picture

MEET WALTER BRYANT:

I'd like to introduce you to one of our favourite therapy clients. I know we're not supposed to have favourites, but if not for Walter, I'm not sure that we'd be as popular as we are today. This is the story of how we met. I'll give you my version and then I'll give you Walter's family's version.

I received an email from a friend who works at our local Alzheimer's Society, explaining that she had been working with a family whose father might benefit from my dog therapy and asking if she could pass on my info. Of course, I replied.

After speaking with his family, I was under the impression that the father, Walter, had been moved into a nursing home and since then had declined considerably. He wasn't communicating well. He wasn't enjoying life at all. He had lost his zest for living. We talked about Walter's past, and it came to light that he had always had dogs, so when his daughter-in-law asked me if I thought that he could benefit from this kind of program, my answer was simply, "Well, it can't hurt right? Let's give it a shot."

We set a date and for the first visit I decided it would be best to only come with one dog. That would be my superstar, Harold.

We were waiting around the corner for Walter and his daughter-in-law, Chris, in the lounge area, and when she wheeled Walter around that

Lucky's Way

corner…BAM…Walter lit right up! He looked right at Harold, and with a huge smile on his face said, "There he is! Come here, Tiger! Look at him!"

That was it! It was love at first sight for both of them. On that very first visit, they made a connection. It was so amazing to witness. It doesn't happen often, but when it does, it hits me right in my heart and it makes my heart smile for a long time!

Soon more and more patients came out of their rooms to visit with Harold. Then something very interesting happened. Suddenly, Harold pulled me over to Walter and methodically straddled Walter's wheelchair. He did it in slow motion so as not to step where he shouldn't and then stood there. I had never seen him do this before, so I have to admit that I was feeling a little nervous, not really knowing what he was doing. I tried to pull him away, but Harold stood stock still and wouldn't budge.

I noticed that he was very intensely watching this gentleman who was helping another woman out of the nursing home to a vehicle. Harold kept watching until that car pulled away and then he slowly backed up and backed off Walter's wheelchair.

Thankfully, my friend Lizzy was there to witness this as well. I get to see all kinds of wonderful and amazing things that my dogs do when it comes to helping people, but having someone else witness protective behaviour like this, well, that's just awesome! To this day I can't explain why Harold felt he needed to protect Walter. He just did. I can't explain a lot of things that my therapy dogs do out of sheer instinct. That's what makes them AWESOME!

Walter has since moved nursing homes, so we moved with him! We still keep the same schedule at his old nursing home, but now we visit Walter and bringing our dog therapy team to his new home and his new friends. Needless to say, thanks to Walter, in his new home they now have a dog therapy program on their regular schedule.

The funniest thing happened on one of our visits. We showed up and I asked the PSW (Personal Support Worker) where Walter was. It happened to be the day that I had brought along my photographer to take pictures for this book and I specifically wanted pictures of Walter and Harold.

She told me that he wasn't feeling up to coming to group today. I smiled, knowing Walter well, and said to her, "Here, take Harold with you. I guarantee you he'll come down then." The PSW stood there with a very unconvinced look on her face. I decided to go over her head and I simply said the magic words to Harold: "Go find your friend Walter, Harold…go find him, go on, go get Walter!" and he took off down the hall, PSW in tow.

Nancy French, my photographer, jumped up, saying, "I have to follow along and see what happens next! I just have to! Is that okay, Brenda?"

"Sure," I said, "but I know Walter and he's going to come down to see the dogs."

It was only a matter of minutes before I saw the PSW, Harold, Nancy, and Walter coming back down the hallway. Walter was darn near jogging to keep up with Harold, and calling after Harold, "Slow down, Charlie, you know I can't walk that fast anymore!" But he was just beaming! Absolutely smiling ear to ear. (Some of my Alzheimer's clients call my dogs by the names of dogs from their own past…Charlie, Fritz, Molly, Emma…it doesn't matter, my boys don't care, they just take it all in stride.)

All of my boys adore Walter. They all rush over to see him and they get very jealous of each other. It's so cute. Harold is definitely the worst for being jealous. He'll try to climb up onto the chair with Walter and Walter just laughs and laughs. Meanwhile, I'm freaking out, thinking that the chair's going to fall over or poor Walter is going to get squished or something. But Walter just tells me, "Leave them be. They're fine. Just leave them alone; they just all want a turn to be pet, don't you, Tiger?" and that's it, that's what it's like when they see Walter.

By the way, did I mention Walter happens to be ninety-three years young? Yes, he's amazing! Close to seven hundred pounds of dogs mauling this adorable ninety-three-year-old gentleman and he's telling me to "leave them alone!" What a gentleman. No wonder he's one of our favourites, eh?

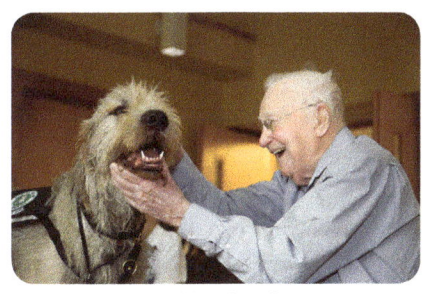

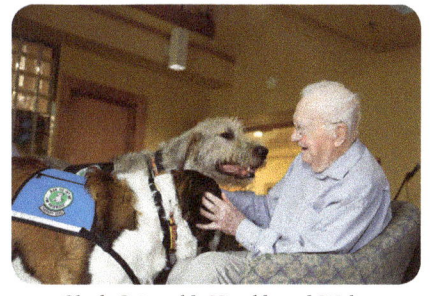

Harold and Walter

Clark Griswald, Harold, and Walter

From the family of Walter Bryant:

We first heard of Brenda and GG Therapy Dogs when we went to the Alzheimer's Society in Stratford looking for support for Walter Bryant.

Walter was dealing with Alzheimer's and, like many families, we were concerned about his day-to-day routines. He rarely socialized in his long-term-care facility and spent most of the day in his room. Even with encouragement he opted out of the planned events.

We made contact with Brenda and set up a visit. She arrived with Harold alone the first time. The expression on Walter's face when he saw Harold was priceless. We had not seen him that happy and excited for years. It was as if Harold was his own dog.

Over time Brenda brought more dogs and it has continued to be the best thing for Walter (and other residents). He almost runs down the hall when he sees the dogs.

In turn, the dogs have really taken to Walter. Our family cannot thank Brenda enough for volunteering her time with the residents. We see the joy she brings, and will always be grateful to her. She's brought a ray of sunshine into Walter's soul.

Brenda Boemer-Groenestege

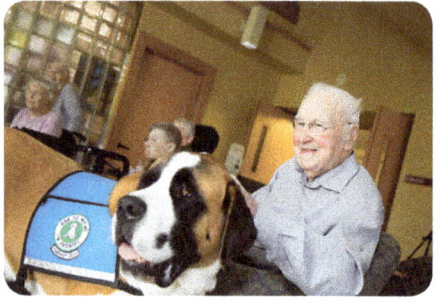

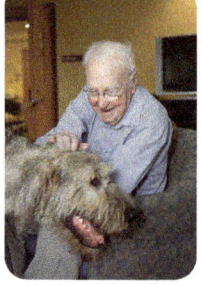

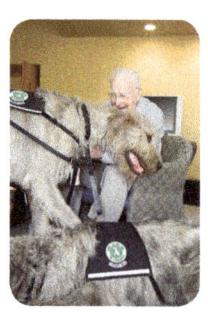

Lloyd and Walter *Harold and Walter* *Walter, Harold, and Leonard*

There are a few other favourite people; actually, there are so many that I can't list them all, but here are a few pictures. As the saying goes, a picture is worth a thousand words.

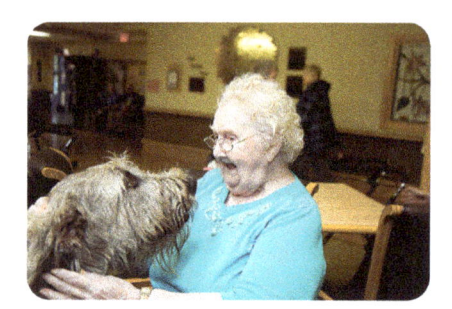

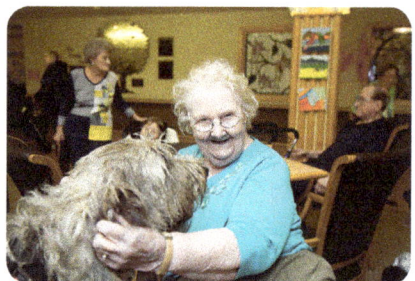

Jean welcomes the love from Harold...

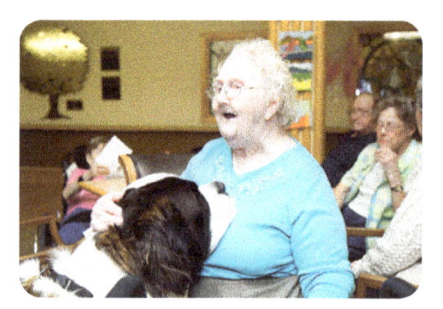

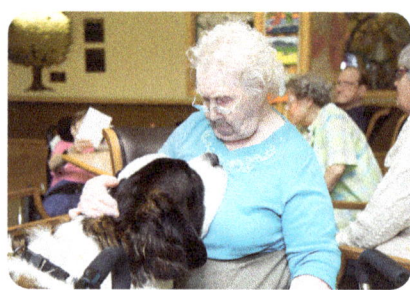

and Clark Griswald absolutely adores Jean

Lucky's Way

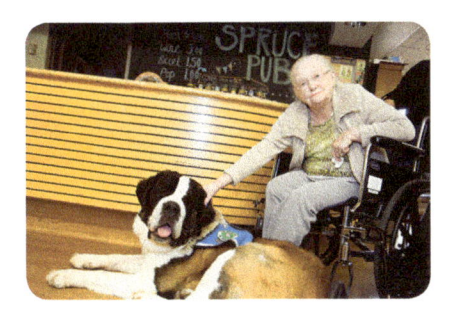

Clark Griswald and Jean

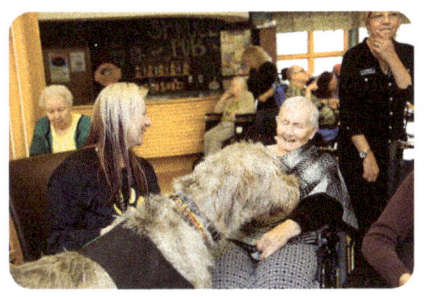

Harold and Johanna, aka Gramma

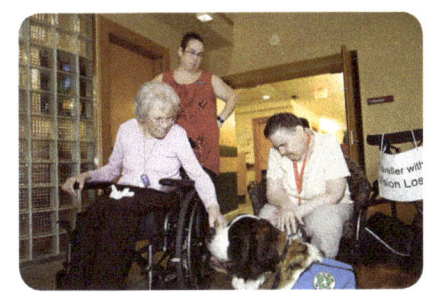

Clark and Janet

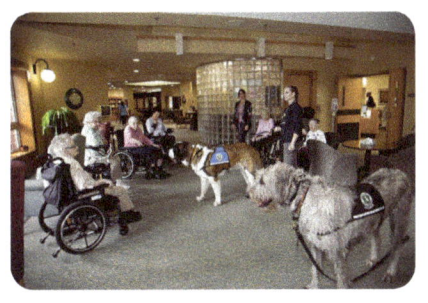

Group therapy at Greenwood Court Stratford

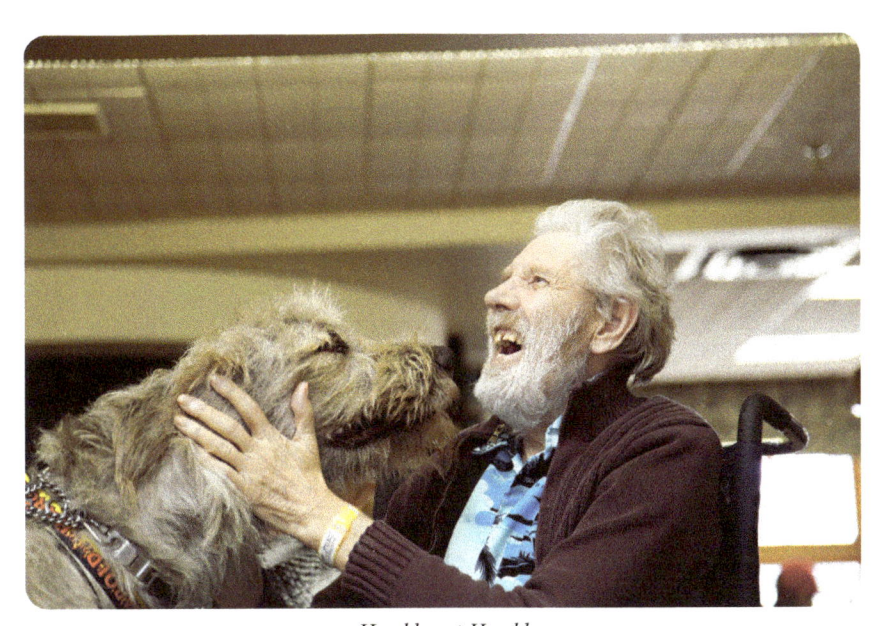

Harold meet Harold

Brenda Boemer-Groenestege

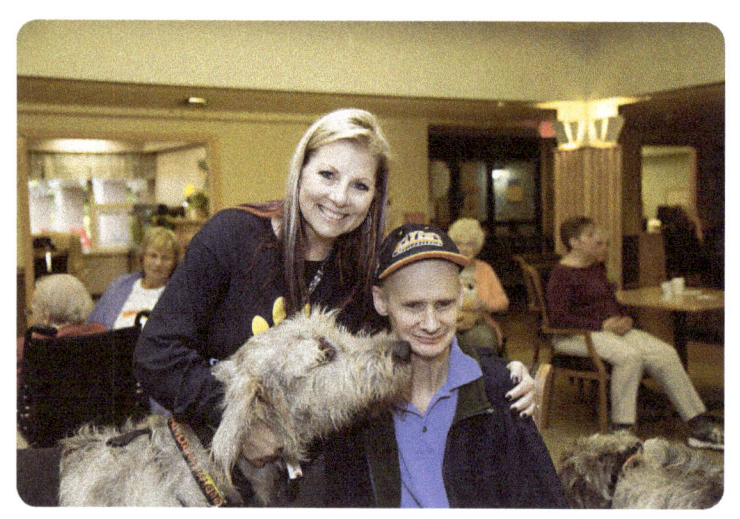

Steven

Steven was another of the dogs' favourite people. Every time we would get to the Spruce Lodge in Stratford, Steven would be waiting for us at the front door. He was always my helper and it was very much appreciated.

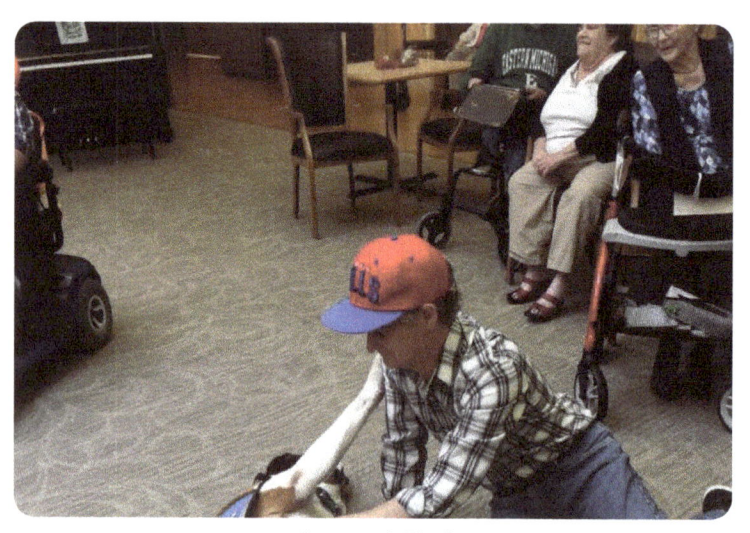

Steven with Lloyd

Over the winter, Steven took a turn for the worse, and stopped meeting us. He then stopped coming to group therapy as well, so we would have to go find him.

Lucky's Way

It got really scary because, as you know, the dogs can sense when people are feeling down. So, when we would go visit Steven and he would be sleeping, my dogs would give him tiny kisses to wake him up.

Now, kissing is absolutely forbidden in my books! It's something that I've trained each of my dogs NOT to do, so for them to go up to Steven and give him a little kiss on the tip of his nose, well, it not only surprised Steven, but it shocked the heck out of me too.

Slowly, though, Steven had begun to feel a bit better, and when we showed up with our photographer for pictures, well, let's just say it was excitement overload when the dogs saw Steven walk into group therapy. They absolutely bombarded him!

Thankfully, a quick-minded PSW grabbed a chair and we got Steven in a chair before the dogs knocked him to the ground and laid a good loving on him.

The smile on Steven's face…well, let's just say it was priceless! There were nurses, volunteers, and staff in tears watching what was happening. I quite often say, "You can't train that into a dog…that just comes naturally," and when it came to Steven, well, my boys very naturally loved him. The feeling was definitely mutual. Before Steven got sick, he would get right down on the floor with the dogs and give them belly rubs and loving. Dogs don't ever forget kindness.

Sadly, we lost Steven in the winter of 2018. He was very special to me as well as my dogs, and he is missed. I will never forget him.

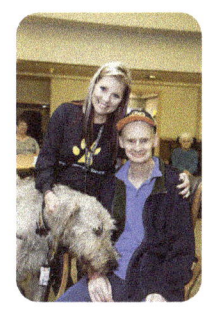

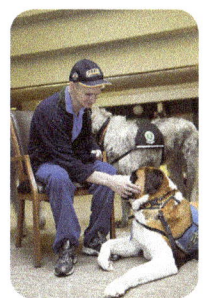

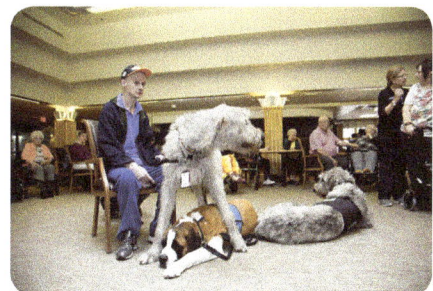

Harold, Steven, and me

This was a really great day. Lloyd and Leonard joined in.

AUDREY

This little lady has stolen not only my heart, but Harold's as well.

I've been taking the boys to the Ritz Lutheran Villa nursing home for about a year and a half. Audrey would come to group therapy every time with her legs crossed and pulled up, her arms folded over her chest, and one hand over her face. Pretty much covering her entire face.

She would always have a really bitter look on her face. She looked like she was angry at the world. If one of the dogs got too close, she would scream, "Get out of here!" Some days she would add an extra word or two and say, "Get the hell out of here! I don't want that dog near me!" So I'd apologize to her and pull them away.

I remember distinctly that it was Valentine's Day, 2018, and Audrey looked just as disgruntled as ever. Harold walked over beside her and when she wasn't paying attention, he very quickly, but super gently, gave her a tiny little kiss on the very tip of her nose!

I couldn't believe he did that. Of all the dogs, he's by far the best trained, so he NEVER ever kisses people!

Well, Audrey was shocked! She sat there with her mouth gaping open and her eyes as wide as saucers!

I looked at her and said, really loudly, "Oh my goodness! Did Harold just give you a kiss? I can't believe that! He only kisses the prettiest girl in the room! That sneaky boy! Well, he sure is right though. He kissed a really pretty girl!"

Audrey didn't know what to say. She just looked at me, then looked at Harold, and sat there, stunned.

I quickly added, "Oh, you better watch him; now that he's kissed you once, he may just try to sneak another kiss, that silly boy."

Well, Audrey wouldn't take her eyes off Harold the entire hour that we were there. It was so funny.

The next time we went in, what did Harold do? Well, if the little bugger doesn't go over, stand right beside Audrey's wheelchair, and when she's not looking, gives her a quick kiss on her nose again.

This time Audrey squealed, "He did it again!"

I jumped. "No way! He kissed the prettiest girl in the room again?"

Lucky's Way

This time, I saw the little smile on Audrey's face. Unbelievable. She was still sitting the same way, all closed off, but she kept an eye on Harold the whole time.

Okay, fast forward to the present…now when we go in, she's all smiles, nudging her neighbours and saying, "Watch out for him, watch out for Harold! He'll sneak a kiss when you're not looking! He's a sneaky one, he is!" And darn it all, if Harold doesn't go over, stand beside her wheelchair, pretend to completely ignore her, and when she's not paying attention, lean over and give her a little kiss.

We have this on video, and it's so amazing to watch. Audrey squeals in delight and if Harold could strut, well, that's what he would do. Again, you can't train that into a dog! That is something that comes so naturally to him. And that's why I call Harold my superstar.

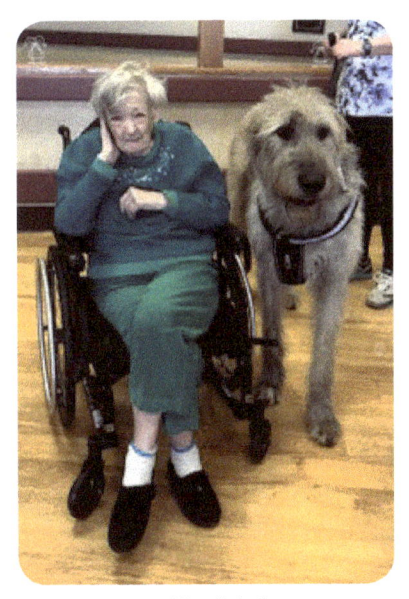

Harold and Audrey

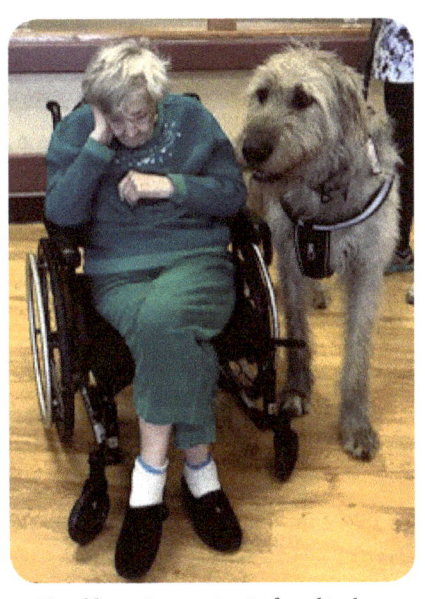

Harold was just moving in for a kiss here.

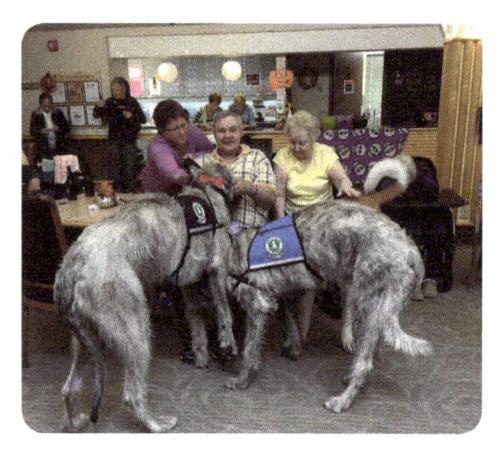

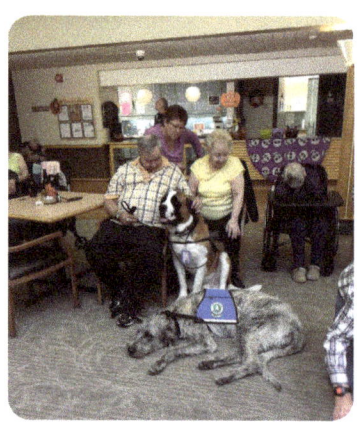

WALTER BRYDGES

Another very special man from therapy was Walter Brydges. The dogs look forward to seeing certain people when we go into places and Walter was definitely one of those people.

Walter was sight-impaired, so he always appreciated how wonderful my boys smelled (because of the Moroccan-oil that I use on them) as well as how soft they were. Walter's favourite dog was Clark Griswald. He loved the fact that when I first brought Clark into where Walter lived, he could sit on his lap, but within a year, Clark had gotten to be 165 pounds of fluffy awesomeness!

When we went to visit in December 2018, just before Christmas, I was approached outside by Walter's friend Kim, who informed me that Walter had suddenly passed away, peacefully, just a few days before. She thanked us for all the joy we had brought Walter, because he had absolutely loved and looked forward to our visits. We miss Walter.

There is another lovely lady we visit regularly in one of the nursing homes, and her name is Mona. The first time we visited her was because she was calling for help! She was calling and calling repeatedly for help, and Harold heard her and immediately dragged me to her. I was very proud of him for being so attentive. Mona doesn't actually need help, she just cries out for it all the time. That's how she communicates right now. It can be very confusing for Harold. Sometimes we just sit with her and I hold her hand until she falls asleep. If we try to carry on with our room to room visits while Mona is calling out for help, it just doesn't work because Harold keeps pulling me back to check on Mona. On our last visit with Mona, I came to find out that when we visit, she's so happy that it's one of the only times people hear her talking in complete sentences. Now that makes us feel good. And Mona loves it when she gets to hold Harold's leash while I push her wheelchair up and down the hall in the nursing home. She's such a sweet lady.

Another one of our favourite people to visit is Henriette. She and I have a special connection because of my middle name (Henrietta), so we call ourselves the "trouble twosome" and she thinks that's just so funny. She will walk with me and my dogs down the hall and sometimes she forgets where her room is, so we find it together. By the time we get back to her room, she's happy to just rest in her easy chair, so she leans on Harold for support and eases herself down. Then Henriette will giggle away because she thinks it's so funny that she used a dog to lean on. When we say goodbye, she will get upset for a minute, because she knows that we won't see each other for a few weeks. It really is a special bond that we've created.

Next is Joan. Now, this wonderful woman and Harold go way back. We first met Joan when she was in the hospital and we were doing our rounds. Harold was just a young pup, and still very much in training, and when he got beside Joan's bed, he decided to get up on it and straddle her! She cried out in pain! OH MY LORD! I felt awful! I apologized over and over again, and after I found out that the lady was okay, we left the hospital. Now, two years later, here she is, in one of the nursing homes that we visit regularly. She's one of the sweetest and funniest women that we visit. She loves to tell the story of how her and Harold first met, much to my chagrin, but she says that she was the crybaby back then. I adore her, and so do my dogs.

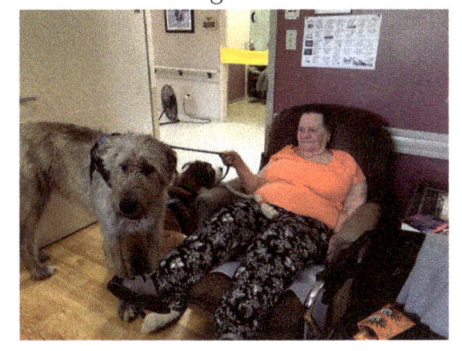

Brenda Boemer-Groenestege

Sometimes the dogs and I may be the only visitors that some people get in the nursing homes or hospitals, sadly enough. It's something that I never realized until I started doing this kind of work. The gratitude that people show is unbelievable. Having a visit from a therapy dog for five, ten, fifteen minutes means the world to these people. It truly is a rewarding job.

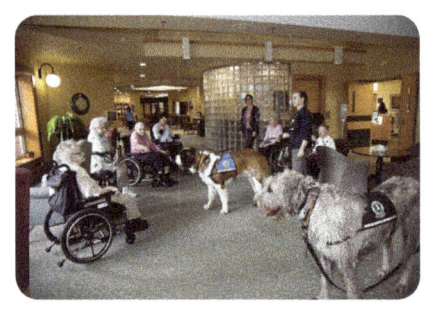

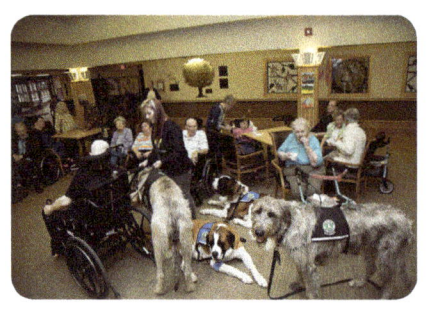

Group Therapy at Greenwood

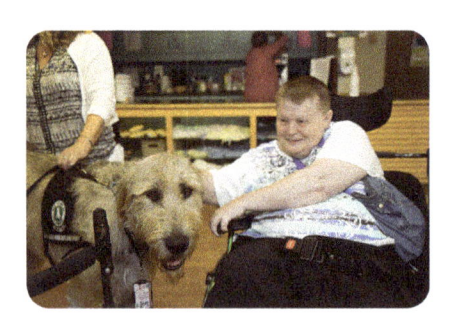

Harold & Darlene

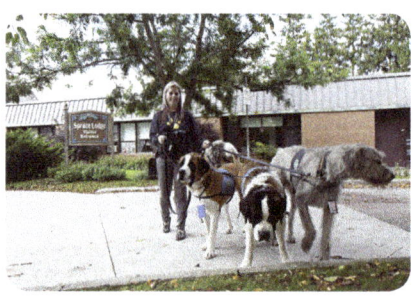

Leaving Spruce Lodge

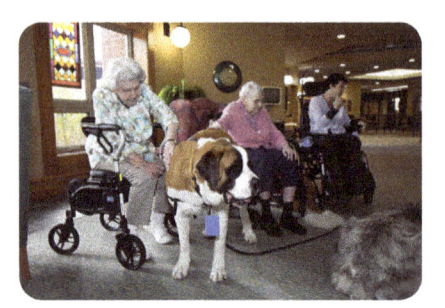

Lloyd is rockin' group therapy

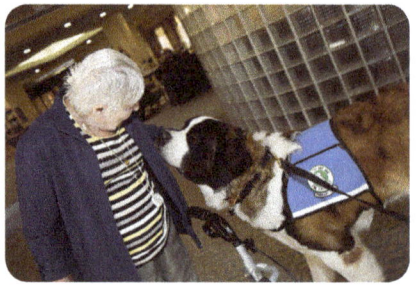

Shirley and Clark Griswald. I've known Shirley since I was fifteen years old.

Lucky's Way

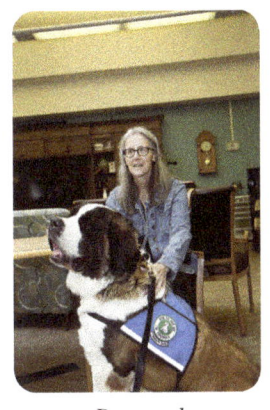

*Darcy and
Clark Griswald*

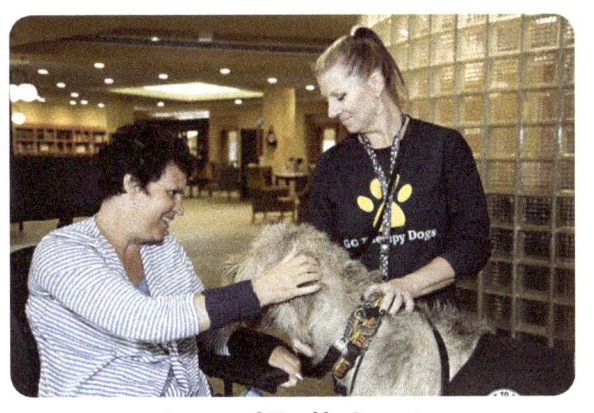

*Joanne and Harold... Joanne is
another major dog lover!*

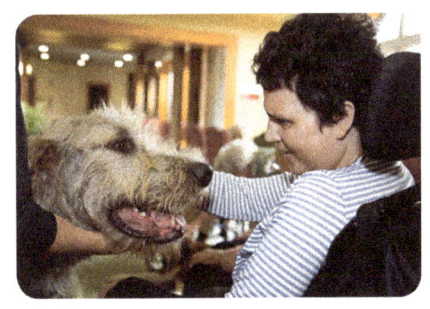

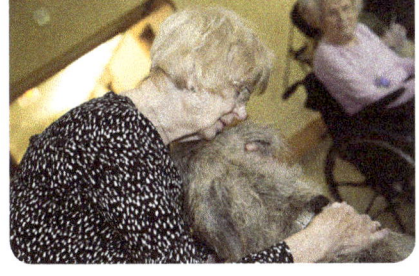

*In this picture, I'm holding Harold back from climbing onto
Joanne's wheelchair...not that she would mind.*

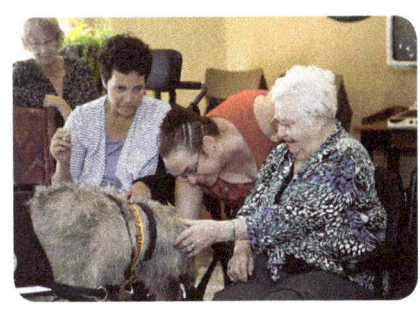

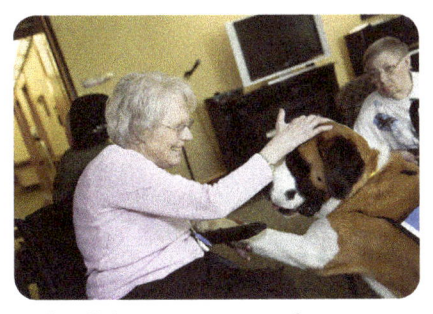

Watching the adoration exchanged between dogs & humans is very rewarding

CHAPTER 11

All Good Things Must Come To an End

THAT DAMN RAINBOW BRIDGE

I've been dreading having to write this chapter for a long time. Unfortunately, it's an inevitable part of life that we, as humans, will lose our pets either to old age or to humane euthanasia because of sickness or an accident. Either way (as my husband says to me when I go through this), we are supposed to outlive our pets.

It doesn't make it any easier, does it? It's still such a difficult and heart-wrenching thing when we lose a pet because they really are a part of our family. For some of us, they are a very, very big part of our family.

Okay, so how do you decide when it's the "right" time to say goodbye to your pet?

Well, if your dog has joint issues like my old Saint Bernard Truman did, this is what my vet, Dr. Angela, said: "If you have a large or giant breed of dog and he or she cannot walk up or down the stairs on their own, it's time to let them go." That's as straightforward as it gets.

In smaller breeds, it's harder to pinpoint one definite obvious sign. Especially since the small breeds tend to live quite a long life.

My BFF, Julie, and my brother Joe had a Jack Russell/poodle mix. Her name was Reggie. Personally, I prefer my giant breeds over the little toy breed dogs, but Reggie stole my heart from day one. She was awesome! She was one of those dogs who looked in the mirror and saw a Great Dane in the reflection. She was tough as nails. It didn't matter how big the other dog was, Reggie could and would try to take em' on! At the end, we all called her "Zombie Dog" because she was blind, deaf, and had maybe five teeth left, but other than that, she was a pretty healthy seventeen-year-old dog.

Do you know that, given a chance, your dog would wander away and find somewhere to die if you let it? But of course we would never let that happen because we watch them like hawks, or at least I do, when they are old and feeble.

Truman would quite often try to wander off at the end but I would be outside, in the middle of the night, in my pjs, slippers, and housecoat, with a flashlight, roaming the property looking for him. Was he happy to see me when I found him? I always thought so, but he was probably actually thinking, "Good God, lady, leave me the hell alone! I just want some damn peace! Do you seriously have to follow me everywhere? What is wrong with you?"

Then what do we do? We get electric fencing installed to keep the dogs in. I'm not even going to imagine what Truman would have begun to think of me for that nonsense!

When Truman stopped being able to do the stairs on his own, that's when I made the decision for him. We still miss him every day, of course.

How do you decide if your dog *isn't* old? What if your dog is dangerous? How do you know when it's time to make that phone call to your vet?

I told you I would finish Bud's story, and this is how it goes...

Since the day I brought Earl home, it was a power struggle between him and Bud. They just didn't like each other. The older Earl got, the more volatile the situation got between them. It seemed like a jealousy issue at first, but soon enough I realized that it was a full-on battle over who was going to be the alpha dog.

Even though I like to think *I'm* the pack leader, there is still a definite hierarchy amongst the dogs. Bud, being the oldest, would always want to claim or fight for dominance, but Earl was progressively becoming more mature and stronger and was challenging Bud every chance he got.

On this particular day, it was a beautiful cool, crisp fall morning and Earl and I had just delivered coffee and muffins to Bob and the guys at the job site. Bob had given me strict instructions for that day: they were putting the roof trusses on the shop they were building, it was going to be an all-hands-on-deck situation and a *do not disturb him* kind of day.

I got the message loud and clear. I remember, as I was leaving the job site, my son Dylan, who was working for us at the time, gave me a knowing wink after he heard his dad say this to me. We all knew what it meant when Bob said he didn't want to be disturbed. No phone calls, no text messages, no nothing! Gotcha! With a quick wave, Earl and I headed home.

As soon as I got home, I opened the back hatch of my SUV to let Earl jump out, and before I even had a chance to turn around, BAM, Bud was on him and the fight of all fights began!

Now, in the back of my mind, I could hear César Millán saying, "Remain calm, you can't panic or it will escalate the situation." I took a deep breath, walked over, grabbed each of them by the collar, and started pulling them apart. The whole time I was yelling, "OFF, STOP, OFF!"

All of a sudden, Bud let go of Earl and turned on me. He grabbed hold of my right forearm and hung on. I was screaming in pain.

I noticed that his eyes had gone completely blank. It was like he wasn't even there. I tried to pry open his mouth but I couldn't. Finally Earl came running over and grabbed Bud by the throat and he released me.

Bugger, bugger, bugger! I had blood pouring out of my arm. I ran into the house, pulled up my sleeve, and started running water on the cut. I saw the water going in one hole and out the other side of my arm. Oh crap. If there's one thing I just can't handle it's my own blood.

I quickly opened the bottom drawer in the bathroom where I keep our animal first aid kit and wrapped my arm in vet wrap to stop the bleeding. The next big problem was that I was on the verge of passing out.

Again, crap! I didn't know what to do. Luckily, our cordless phone had been left on the vanity in the bathroom, so I grabbed it, crawled to the kitchen and lay down on the floor so I didn't pass out and called 911.

"What is your emergency?" the operator asked.

"I was bitten on the arm by my dog," I told her, "and I'm about to pass out."

"Okay, just stay with me; where is your dog now?" she asked.

Well, then I had to explain the whole story and that he's not vicious to people, he just got in a fight with my other dog, and stupid me thought I could break it up.

"Is there someone else there who can lock the dogs up before the ambulance gets there?" she asked.

"No, my husband's working and he's really busy and I'd really rather not call him unless it's really important," I explained.

"Umm, Brenda, you've been bitten by your dog and an ambulance is en route. Do you not think this constitutes important?" she asked, somewhat sarcastically.

Ah, crap. "Fine" I said, very disgruntled, "I'll call him but he's going to be really mad at me." I hung up the phone and called Bob.

"Yes, what?" he answered.

"Hi babe, umm, listen, don't rush or anything, but the dogs got into a fight again and when I tried to break them up, Bud bit me pretty bad. I'm lying on the floor in the kitchen and I really didn't want to bug you because I know how busy you are but the 911 operator made me call you 'cause the ambulance is coming and she's afraid the dogs might bite them or something stupid. She just wants you to lock them up and then you can go back to work, okay? I'm really sorry, Bob." There was nothing on the other end of the phone when I was done talking. Well, crap again. "Bob? Hello? Bob?"

He had hung up on me since he had jumped into his truck and was screaming home.

I heard the ambulance and then the police and finally Bob pulled in too. I could hear them yelling because the doors were all open.

Policeman: "Sir, if you don't get control of your dogs I'm going to have to shoot them!"

Bob: "Good! Shoot them! Shoot every f'n one of them! Do it! You'd be doing me a favour!"

Policeman: "Sir, please, control your dogs!"

Bob: "They're not my f'n dogs! They're my wife's! Just shoot them! Shoot them all!"

Me: "DON'T YOU DARE SHOOT MY DOGS! I SWEAR I'LL SHOOT YOU!"

Lucky's Way

EMT: "Ma'am, you have to lie still and let us do our job, please. Getting upset will only make things worse."

Me: "IF YOU SHOOT MY DOGS I SWEAR TO GOD THERE'LL BE HELL TO PAY!"

EMT: "Please, Brenda."

Policeman: "Sir, I can't shoot your dogs. You just have to lock them in the garage."

Bob: "Fine. Stupid f'n animals. I never wanted them in the first place!"

With the dogs safely locked away, they loaded me in the ambulance and took me to the hospital. I had to get multiple layers of stitches to close the wound but there was no permanent damage.

By the time I got back home, Bud's fate had already been sealed. I was heartbroken. When I looked back at the last year of Bud's life, however, I realized that he had changed drastically, I just hadn't wanted to see it. He had been on daily pain medication for his joints, and there were days that he was having trouble walking because of stiffness.

No one except me was willing to feed him because he was being unpredictable around food. That should have set off warning signals for me, but I guess I just didn't want to hear it. He was my last tie to my dad and I wanted to hold onto that for as long as possible. Every time I looked at Bud, I remembered what my dad said…"That's the best dog she's ever going to have," and it made me feel so good.

I have so many really amazing memories of him, and he really was the best dog ever. I'm thankful that it was me he bit and not someone else because I could never have forgiven myself if that was the case.

That brings me too Earl. We think Earl was progressively going blind. This is very difficult to diagnose in a dog without taking him to a university-level veterinary clinic, which specializes in those types of things.

Besides, Earl was always the type of dog that one might consider a loose cannon of sorts. One that you couldn't always trust around other dogs or people, so that put us on edge constantly. We run a business out of our home and we are constantly getting deliveries to our house. For the first two years or so, it was okay, but then we started getting complaints that our dog was being aggressive and the delivery drivers were afraid to get out of their trucks. That was not okay.

To be completely honest, I thought they were being a little bit overly dramatic in their accusations. When I was home, Earl was such a sweetheart that I had a hard time believing that he could be so vicious. However, as a responsible dog owner, I thought I had better deal with this quickly and forcibly. Not as easy as I thought it was going to be.

I tried, quite literally, everything from stern voice commands to a remote shock collar. I even got him neutered at an earlier age than I'd hoped in order to suppress his testosterone levels, and I have to confess that I was feeling quite defeated. Earl was not responding to any training techniques. It was a real head-scratcher.

Then, one day when Brooklyn got off the school bus, I was outside with Earl and Truman, and Earl took off barking like a mad dog, heading toward Brooklyn! His hackles were up from the tip of his tail to the top of his head and he was snarling like she was coming at us like an ax murderer! It was absolutely shocking to witness.

Brooklyn stopped in her tracks and called out to him, "Earl, it's me, what are you doing, buddy?" And just like that, his whole demeanour changed and he was super sweet and loving again. As soon as he heard her voice, he obviously recognized her and then all was good. Had I not seen it with my own eyes, I truly think I would not have believed it.

That same day, we received our brand new John Deere tractor. Needless to say, there was quite a bit of excitement around our house. My husband and our boys were super excited about it and some of the neighbours also stopped in to check it out.

Coincidentally, the neighbour girl next door biked over to see Brooklyn at the very same time as all the commotion was going on with the shiny, new tractor.

I had Earl on a leash because I wasn't sure how he was going to react with all the people, and the delivery truck and so forth, but then I eventually took the leash off. That's when he did the strangest thing. Ultimately, the thing that signed his death certificate.

The neighbour girl was simply talking to Brooklyn while casually sitting on her bike when Earl walked in a circle around the two girls twice, then turned, looked directly at me, making full eye contact, before turning back and grabbing the sleeve of the girl's sweatshirt.

I couldn't believe my eyes! I ran over to her and asked if she was okay. And she said yes, that he had just grabbed her sleeve. I made her show me her arm to make sure, and I didn't see any marks at all, thank God.

To this day it still shakes me up when I think of that. I keep seeing him looking directly at me before he did it, like he was trying to tell me something. Is that possible?

I walked him into the house, where I completely broke down and lost my composure. After I pulled myself together, I called my vet clinic and made an appointment for the next day to put him down.

That was a very tough twenty-four hours to go through. I kept asking Earl, why? Not that I expected an answer from him, but I just didn't understand.

He was only three years old and no matter how ugly some people thought he was, I thought he was beautiful. No matter how vicious he could be, he was always sweet me. No matter how dumb certain family members claimed him to be, he always came through in emergency situations. Most of all, no matter what anyone else thought, I loved him with my whole heart and I know he loved me back, unconditionally.

While I was driving to the vet clinic, I was second-guessing myself. I just wasn't sure if putting him down was absolutely necessary. I turned to prayer for guidance, as I often do, and I asked God to send me a sign of some sort, just to let me know if I was doing the right thing.

Just then, a beautiful beam of sunshine showed up directly in front of my car and quite literally stayed there the entire trip to the vet clinic. I took that as my sign.

There was a song by Bruno Mars playing in my truck, the one that goes, "You're simply amazing just the way you are." That's how I felt about Earl. I looked into my rearview mirror and saw him sitting there, just as content as can be. Just this big goofy black and white dog who I loved dearly. I know a lot of people didn't like him, but it didn't matter because *I* loved him. He was *my* sweet boy and he was always there for me. I miss him dearly too.

I have lost dogs through accidents on the road or because of other matters out of my control, and it always hurts when they cross over that damn rainbow bridge. It doesn't matter if you've had that pet for ten days or ten years; if we lose them, it hurts and we grieve. My only consolation is that I know they're all up there hanging out with my dad. Now that makes me smile.

We connect with our pets immediately, and most of the time the feeling is mutual. It may take a day or two after you first get your puppy or your rescue dog before you notice the connection, but if *you* are all in, I guarantee you that your furry pal will give you one hundred percent! That's the beauty of dogs; they don't know how to half-ass things. They are always fully committed! They are always all in!

Because of this kind of commitment that we've given to our pets and they've given back to us, I understand it is very hard to make the choice to humanely euthanize your furry pal, but I ask you, Would you want to go through life, possibly in excruciating pain but not being able to verbalize it? What if there was a way to end your suffering and just painlessly fall asleep? I know the choice I would make, if I could make it.

This is when we should always rely on our vets to be completely honest with us as to how much pain our beloved pet is in. Ask them, "Am I keeping my pet alive just for me?"

But then you must be prepared to *HEAR* the true answer.

When it became clear that Truman could no longer hold up his hind end very well, I rushed him in to see the vet. I guess I knew what the answer was going to be, but hearing her say that it was time for us to consider putting him down was still very difficult.

Especially Truman, everyone loved Truman. He was always so sweet-natured and loving, and *always, always* there for anyone who was feeling down. Truman never once had a bad day, or if he did, he certainly didn't show it. He was my original therapy dog and I wasn't even in the business yet. Family, friends, neighbours…anyone who knew Truman knew how much love he gave every day and to everyone. It was instinctual with him. If you were sick, or upset, maybe just had a fight with your husband or your parents, or you had a bad day at school, whatever the problem, Truman would instinctively come over to you and lie right on your feet,

Lucky's Way

or he'd sit and keep lifting one paw because he wanted to hold hands with you.

Some people would just show up needing their Truman time. My niece Yvonne for example, had a very special connection with Truman. When that girl came over, he would not leave her alone! From the minute she pulled in the driveway, he would run to her and that was it, she was stuck with him! Not that Yvonne minded. She would sometimes sleep over and he slept right beside her, making sure she was okay.

There were times when we would visit her at work. Coincidentally, Yvonne worked at the senior living community where my mom lives, and if I wasn't paying attention, Truman would catch a glimpse of his buddy Yvonne and BAM, like a shot, he was gone, and I was dragging behind him. He just had to get to her. It really was quite a thing to witness. She has a special connection with all my dogs, but she just seemed to have that extra soft spot in her heart for Truman.

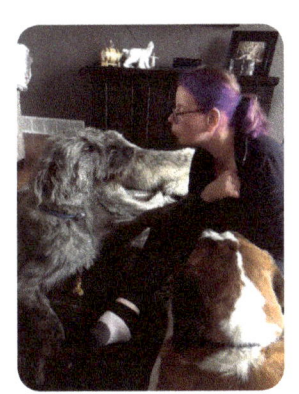

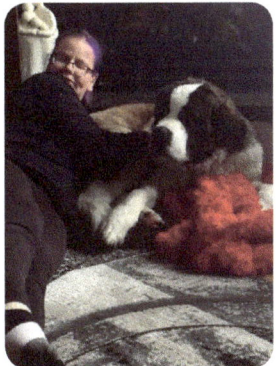

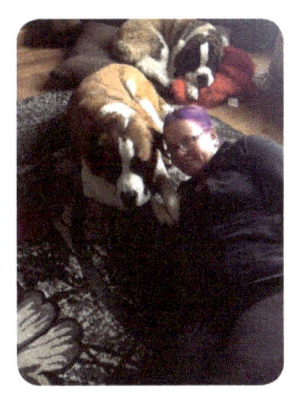

Yvonne with Leonard, Clark Griswald, and Lloyd

Truman would do the silliest thing every day: he would all of a sudden just start to wind up and begin barking, slowly at first, until it turned into a howl! Of course, that would get all the other dogs in the house, whether they lived here or were just visiting, howling as well. It would drive Bob bananas!

After hearing the bad news, I told Dr. Angela that I had to give my family a chance to say goodbye to him and she agreed with me completely. Closure is key in these situations.

Bob decided to take the dogs out back for a walk to the bush because it was such a beautiful day. I questioned his judgement on whether Truman should go or not, and then quickly realized that it was Bob who needed the time together, alone with *his* dog. I sometimes forget that some men have different ways of grieving or saying goodbye than what we openly animal lovering people do. It must be terrible feeling like you have to hold that all in?

I heard Bob yelling for me and I ran outside. Truman had lay down on the path on the way back to the house and didn't want to get up. Bob was just yelling at me to bring him a lawn chair so he could sit with Truman until he got up enough strength to walk again.

The next morning I made the phone call to our vet clinic and asked for a home visit to put Truman down. He could no longer do the stairs. I was lifting his hind end up, helping him to walk with a scarf. It was time.

Dr. Angela came right after lunch. Truman was lying down in our garage, and I was, of course, a mess, while Dr. Angela and her assistant (also named Angela) worked on him. Harold had snuck out of the house, and even though I really didn't want him to witness this, he ended up doing the most remarkable thing.

First he had to check every thing out. He began by pulling all the cool stuff out of Dr. Angela's medical bag. Then, he continued by getting into everyone's face and letting them know that he was there for them if they needed him. Finally, as the procedure started, Harold could not seem to settle himself down. I watched him pace back and forth in front of Truman, and just when I was about to put him in the house, he did something really quite remarkable. He stopped, he laid down in front of Truman and began licking Truman's eyes and face. Harold continued to lick Truman's face until he took his very last breath. It was, by far, the most incredible and the sweetest thing I've ever witnessed an animal do and yet the most heartbreaking.

Harold then came over to me and put his head on my lap until I pushed him away because I still needed my time to hug Truman. At that point, he went over to Dr. Angela and gave her some therapy, and then to vet tech Angela, giving her some as well, until he got back to me. Then he wouldn't leave me alone until I got up from the cold garage floor.

Lucky's Way

We all miss Truman. He left a big hole not only in our house, but in a lot of other people's lives too.

However, there is something that makes me think he comes around to visit us daily, or I should say his spirit comes around daily. You see, every day my dogs start to howl! They do the same darn thing that Truman did on a regular basis and I'm convinced that it's Truman's spirit coming to visit us.

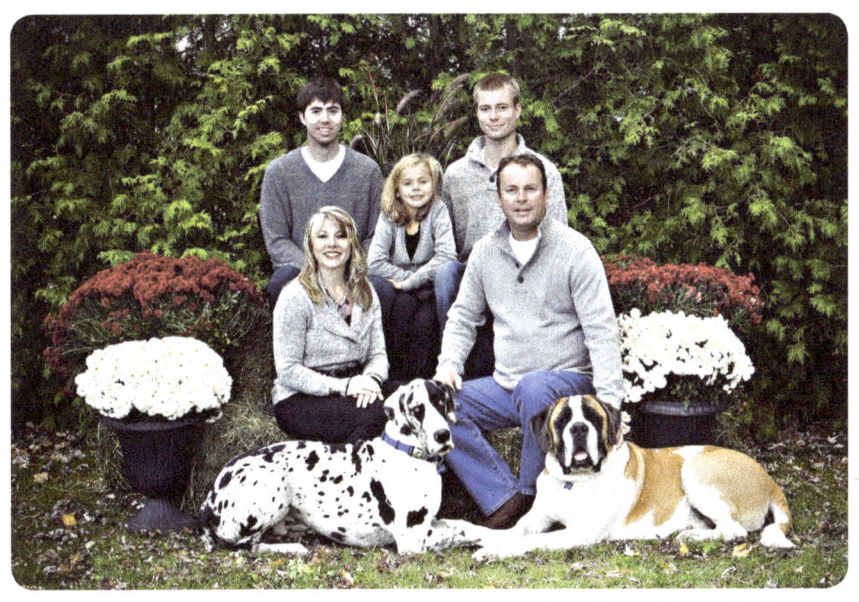

Family portrait taken a few years ago with Truman and Earl. Back row, left to right: Spencer, Brooklyn, and Dylan. Front row: me, Bob, harlequin Great Dane, Earl...Saint Bernard, Truman

CHAPTER 12

Pets Make Us Better People

My pet of choice is obviously a dog, but for others it may be a cat, a horse, a hamster, a rabbit, a bird, a goldfish, a lizard…whatever! It really doesn't matter what kind of pet you have, as long as you love and care for that pet to the best of your ability. And if you're not able to, then do the right thing and find it a good home. No one will judge you for that!

I have had dogs my whole life. They were my very first loves and they will probably be my very last. They understand me in a way that people just don't. They don't seem to think I'm weird or crazy when I'm crying like a baby watching sappy movies on TV or reminiscing about my dad, which brings on the waterworks like Niagara Falls!

Do my dogs judge me? Nope! They don't take one look at me and say, "What the hell is wrong with you now?" and walk out the door without waiting for a response.

The truth is, dogs, or pets for that matter, don't care why you're crying; they just want to be there to make you feel better. They want to be there for you, to lick your tears away, to drape their 185-pound body over your body (thereby damn near crushing you) to show you how much they care about you, to prove to you that they are here for you and that they really do love you unconditionally.

I, for one, can't get enough of that kind of support. When I'm not feeling one hundred percent, all I want is a steaming mug of my favourite green tea, a cosy blanket, a good book, and my dogs. Okay, maybe some good drugs too, depending on the illness (hahaha)!

Seriously, a show of hands, who wants to just be left alone when they're ticked off, upset about something, or not feeling well?

Exactly!

I'm assuming quite a few of you put your hands up! Now, realistically, who actually gets that luxury?

Yes, that's sad, isn't it? Unfortunately, that's why we rely so heavily on our pets, people! Because our everyday, regular life is just a crazy busy gong show and our pets help keep us grounded.

Did you know that the motion of petting your dog or cat actually decreases your blood pressure? That is a scientific fact! You can google that! Walking your dog can decrease the chance of a heart attack! Yes, it can, folks. It gets you in better physical shape, lowers blood pressure, and therefore contributes to better overall body condition: voila, better chance of no heart attack.

Give your dog fifteen minutes of unconditional love and attention before you go to bed at night and I can guarantee it will make you feel less stressed and more relaxed than if you turned on your laptop or iPad or whatever device you're currently addicted to.

I'm going to leave you with this...

Be the person your dog thinks you are...starting right now!

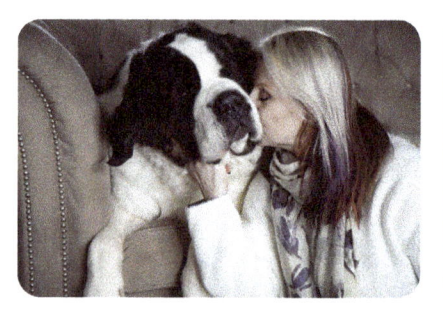

Clark Griswald and me

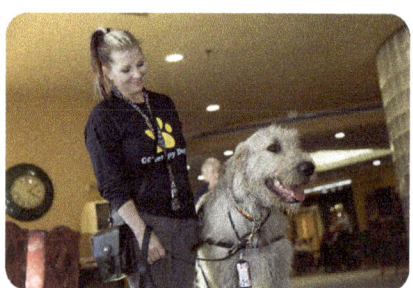

Harold and me

ACKNOWLEDGMENTS

First and foremost I have to thank my daughter Brooklyn. She is not only my number one fan, but she has been my rock as well while writing this book, especially during the editing process. I truly couldn't have made it through without her beside me each step of the way, encouraging me to continuing on when I was ready to throw my laptop through the window. For that, I can't thank her enough. Brooklyn, you really are an incredible source of strength, inspiration and invaluable insight and I hope you know how much I love, respect and treasure, not only you as my daughter, but as an intelligent, beautiful and kind young woman and more importantly, as one of my best friends and closest confidants.

My other sources of inspiration are my sons, Spencer and Dylan. Without them and their ongoing love and support throughout this adventure, again, I don't think this book would have come to fruition. There had been so many times when I was a single mom that I just wanted to give up on life because it was so hard, but my boys kept me going, and for that, I can't thank them enough. They were my biggest challenge, yet always stepped up to prove to be my greatest champions, never leaving me feeling anything but pride for not only them, but their sister as well… who they've stepped in to be her champion as well.

As far as kids go, I really do have the best ones around. They have been amazingly supportive, even when I've been on the verge of losing my shit… they keep me grounded, and help me to see the big picture or book, in this case. Thank you kids, I know I can be a bit of a pain in the ass, but I appreciate it all.

To my friend Lizzy, wow, I don't know where to begin to thank you for everything. Not only are you one of my dearest friends, but you are literally the one person who I always know that I can call on when I need help for anything! You make our house a more beautiful place to come home, and with four big, slobbery, hairy dogs in the house, that's no easy feat. You are, and have always been my number one cheerleader and one of my biggest fans, who continues to encourage me, as well as ensures that I know how much we are appreciated for all the dog therapy visiting that we do. This happens to include her super-sweet 93 year old mother Betty, who lives in one of the nursing homes we visit. If these aren't reasons enough to thank and adore Lizzy, she and her husband Tom are also our dog sitters. They literally move into our house and take the best care possible of my boys; ask any other dog lover, that means the absolute world to me. It means while I'm away, I can actually relax knowing that my fur children are being well cared for. For this, and so much more, I can't express how much we, my family included, love and thank you.

Next, my book would not be the same without the incredible photos that were taken by my amazingly talented photographer and friend, Nancy French. I've known Nancy for close to twenty years and if I had to compare her to something, I'd compare her to a good bottle of wine... she just keeps getting better and better with age. Seriously though Nancy, I can't thank you enough for going over and above (literally - there were times she was standing on a ladder to take a picture), the call of duty, just to get the picture. You are such a beautiful human being, inside and out, and I can't wait to see what our next project will be together... I'm fairly certain it will still contain dogs.

I want to thank all of my German relatives, especially my two uncles, my dad's brother's, Alfons and Franz, for taking the time to sit down with me and share the stories about my dad. I know it's bittersweet talking about him since he's passed away, but I'm hoping that I've made you all proud by honouring his memory with my book. I would also like to thank my mother, who helped me become the person I am today.

I have to thank Nicole Knibbs for all the help she gave me in the computer tech department. I have been hurling obsolescences at my computer for not cooperating with me and if it had not been for Nicole's ongoing patience, I seriously would be replacing both my laptop and my front picture window. I also want to take a minute and thank her for loving my son Spencer in only a way that she knows how. I love him too, so I get it… he is Bob's son after all. I hope you know how much you are loved and appreciated by our whole family, Nicole. Thank you again.

Now I want to take a second to thank everyone who has allowed me the honour of showing their picture in my book. The saying "a picture is worth a thousand words", is such a true statement. I'm not going to individually name everyone right now, I'm just going to say a very big thank you to ALL!

I do have to centre out a few who helped me with the demonstrations in the book. My beautiful niece Jody Jenkins and her two adorable boys, Lincoln and Leo, who were stellar models. They are amazing and I really can't thank them enough.

As well, Ayla and Ryder… you two took my book and turned it into cuteness overload with your pictures! I mean seriously!! There are no words to thank you guys enough for adding your spunk and Ayla, your attitude, that shows in each and every picture. From the bottom of my heart, thank you.

And Emmett, my sweet, sweet Emmett, the pictures of you and Harold are just out of this world! I'm so happy that I get to share such an amazingly funny kid with the rest of the world. I couldn't love you more or thank you enough!

Another thank you has to go out to my vet clinic, Coventry Animal Hospital, and in particular to my friend and vet Dr. Angela Gerretsen and her teams in Stratford and Mitchell. I really don't know what we would do with them. Thank you, thank you, thank you, for everything.

I have to say a huge thank you to my husband Bob for being not only a patient man, but also an unbelievably good provider which has allowed me to do what I'm doing now with my dogs. I appreciate it so, so much, but all of our therapy clients do as well. I also love that he has the complete understanding that in my world, if you make me choose between you and my dogs… you are not going to like the answer!

Thank you to everyone who let me share their story with you, my readers. Without their stories, my book would be just another how-to training manual, but because of all the stories, it's hopefully helped people to understand that we all have crazy in our lives, it's just on a scale of how much and how we handle it.

Brenda Boemer-Groenestege

I have to thank my dogs… without each and every dog, past and present, I wouldn't be the person I am today. I have learned something from each dog that I've ever had the pleasure of loving, but more importantly, they have all taught me something about myself. I certainly wouldn't have the same empathy, the same outlook on life, and most certainly, I wouldn't be going in the same direction that I'm going in in my life right now had it not been for my dogs. They are my life source, my passion and when all is said and done, it's them I look too at the end of the day when I need a shoulder to lean on or cry into, depending on the day.

Last, but certainly not least, I have to thank the man who continues to inspire me everyday to be the person that he was when he was still with us… my dad, Lucky Boemer. Thank you for always being there when I needed you, even if I didn't realize it. Thank you for sharing your love of dogs with me, knowing that by giving me this gift, it was a bond that we shared for the duration of your life and one I carried on, and have passed on, to my own kids. Thank you for being my champion when I needed you the most, and for showing me how to be the kind of parent to my kids that you were to me… sometimes strict, rarely coddled, occasionally harsh, but always directly to the point, never lovey-dovey, but always, always there when needed most. I miss you every day Dad, some days worse than others, but every day nonetheless.

There is one more tidbit I wanted to share with you about my dad. At his funeral, a couple came from hundreds of kilometres aways, they drove for over eight hours in bad weather just to come to a man they had never mets funeral… yes, you read that correctly, they never met my father and here they were, at his funeral. Why? Because, we were told by them, they lived way up north by my dad's hunting camp and years ago when their kids were young, they were very, very poor and one day there was a knock at the door, and there stood this man, a stranger, holding a box filled with a whole butchered pig. But that's not all, they continue, he had brought bags and bags of groceries for them, and even hand-me-down clothing, and toys for their kids. All the while, they told us, our dad never spoke, just shook my husband's hand and drove away. We were in shock! It was like winning the lottery. We had enough food for the whole winter. It took us quite some time to find out who our hero was. But we were told that he did not want any accolades, or anything, he's just a really good man.

Then the woman continued to tell me that as soon as they were able, they started to give back to those in need and it was always in my father's honour. I was so touched.

We heard story after story about dad doing similar things for people. Strangers usually. Dad would hear that someone was in 'need' and the next thing you know, I guess he would show up and deliver. We had people who recognized my dad's picture from the obituaries in the newspaper and they stood, outside, in freezing cold January weather, for hours, just to pay their respects to a man they had never gotten to know his name but... he bought them lunch, or coffee, or helped change a tire, or brought some groceries, or brought bags of clothes etc. it was unbelievable! It was like my dad was living this secret "good guy" life.

I was, have been, and will always be, incredibly proud of my dad for being exactly what we all wish our dad's were... an everyday superhero! I hope that we're making you proud dad, all of us, your kids and grandkids, because you certainly left some big shoes to fill. I love you... we love you, and once again, thank you for sharing all your gifts, and knowledge, with me.

SPECIAL THANKS:
When I decided to self publish my book, I had no idea how much it was going to cost. Around the same time, we were organizing and purging the rooms in our house, so we decided to have a sale and whoever buys something, their name was going to go into the back of my book as a financial contributor. It was a lot of fun and we had a great response.

Special thank you to everyone who contributed including:

Liz Goodyer
Jody Jenkins
Marg VanNynatten
Nicole Knibbs
Victoria Moore
Mallory Anderson-Neeb
Anne Christopoulos
Vanessa Meinen
Victoria Meinen
Vienna Meinen
Lori Meinen
Gerdina Goodyer
Carmen Jenkins
Mellanie Smith
Jess Anderson
Megan Adair

And to those who's names I have forgotten... thank you!

CPSIA information can be obtained
at www.ICGtesting.com
Printed in the USA
BVHW090022231220
595978BV00006B/16